INEVITABLE COLLISION

Warmest wishes &
many thanks!
Tony Williams

INEVITABLE COLLISION

The Inspiring Story That Brought Stem Cell Research to Conservative America

TORY WILLIAMS

Mary Ann Liebert, Inc. publishers

Library of Congress Cataloging-in-Publication Data

Williams, Tory.
Inevitable collision : the inspiring story that brought stem cell research to conservative America / Tory Williams.
pages cm
ISBN 978-1-934854-38-9 — ISBN 978-1-934854-39-6
1. Atchison, T. J.—Health. 2. Embryonic stem cells—Research—United States—History—21st century. 3. Embryonic stem cells—Transplantation—United States. 4. Spinal cord—Wounds and injuries—Treatment—United States. 5. Human embryo—Therapeutic use. I. Reed, Roman, writer of added text. II. Title.
QH588.S83W55 2015
616.02'774—dc23

2014028748

ISBN: 978-1-934854-38-9
ISBN (e-book): 978-1-934854-39-6

Mary Ann Liebert, Inc.
140 Huguenot Street
New Rochelle, NY 10801

Printed in the United States of America.

Miracles come in moments. Be ready and willing.

—Dr. Wayne Dyer

Contents

Literary Disclaimer

This story is told from my perspective and may differ from another. Since beginning this journey in 2010, I have written more than 10,000 pages of notes and recorded over 100 hours of tape from interviews with patients involved in Geron's stem cell clinical trial, their family members and friends, first responders, doctors and nurses from medical facilities where these patients were treated, theologians, scientists, and researchers. I kept a special notebook labeled PRIVILEGED INFORMATION and have returned to these pages often during the last four years. Indeed, the material in this top-secret notebook has been at arm's length, and frequent trips to my safety deposit box have made this quite the adventure.

The standpoint I held early on for *Inevitable Collision* remains grounded to this very day: This is a journey for all people of this world, not mine alone, nor is it a book that preaches or lectures or pushes any religious belief or political viewpoint on the reader. Each page is written in an honest and heartfelt manner to inform you about the extraordinary efforts of patient advocates, scientists, philanthropists, biotech leaders, and researchers from across the globe, and our journey of hope, faith, and courage.

This is a remarkable period in medical history, a stretch of years that our children and grandchildren are certain to hear reference to in classrooms and study halls for decades to come. I have changed only one name in this book to protect the anonymity of this individual, and altered minor details to preserve confidentiality.

—Tory Williams

Prologue: Guys' Night Out

Chatom, Alabama
September 24, 2010

It was just another Friday night lights for young, handsome TJ Atchison. A tank full of gas, a high school football game fifteen miles away from his hometown of Chatom, and plenty of buddies home from college to enjoy the evening with, a young man's trinity; TJ felt certain that it would be an amazing night. He left his mom's home as the late afternoon sun spread across the sky like a friendly arm. TJ smiled as Haleybell and Lucky gave chase in the distance, but his sporty Pontiac G6 was too fast for the family yard dogs.

Tonight, TJ had no idea how drastically his life was about to change. For all he knew, he was attending the biggest game of the year with his pals, the annual grudge match between his alma mater, the Washington County Bulldogs, and the rival Millry Wildcats. Like every other Bulldog fan in the county, there was no sweeter place to be than hanging out with friends watching the most anticipated game of the season.

Indeed, it was a big event for all southwest Alabama football fans. People from every corner of the state made the trip in order to see which team prevailed. With a dozen cars in front of and behind him on the road, TJ made a quick exit off Highway 17 and drove into town to look for his friends. After spotting his tall, lanky cousin filling his Jeep at the Exxon station, TJ pulled his car beside Cameron and parked. Without even a quick hello, he climbed inside the passenger seat and gave a slap on the knee to a friend in the back.

Although the rival match was scheduled to begin at seven o'clock, the parking area at Wildcat Hill was filled well before. With kickoff just thirty minutes away, vehicles were pulling into any available spot on the eight-acre grounds, alongside buses and mud-splattered pickup trucks. Parents, students, and faculty members all moved about the campus, circling one another and calling out both greetings and predictions about the big game. With the car windows rolled down to admit the moist evening air, and the car radio playing loudly, Cameron swung around the sports arena several times before finding a spot near the visitor's section.

As they made their way toward the admissions booth, the place was already electric with excitement—the crowd was standing on its feet doing the wave and cheering loudly as both teams made their way across the field. The Bulldogs welcome was overwhelming. Everywhere TJ looked, he saw a mad sea of maroon and gold banners stabbing the air, and little ones, their team loyalties sewn into their DNA, running around the grandstand with Bulldog tattoos on their faces.

It wasn't long before a spirited roar rose from the Bulldog section of the stadium. At the end of the first quarter, the visiting team was already up by two touchdowns. Watching the game intently from the fence line, TJ was surprised by how quickly the Bulldogs had taken the lead. Far from the nail-biter everyone had anticipated, a rout was taking shape.

Going into halftime with boredom thickening, TJ and his friends talked it over and decided to ride back to Chatom while listening to the remainder of the game on the radio. Shortly after the Bulldog's victory became official, thoughts of an old friend still in the area came to TJ's mind. Impulsively, he scrolled down his phone's contact list and selected Lisa Bradford's number. He intended to ask Lisa if she might be up for a late-night visit.

After pressing "Dial," he immediately felt unsure of himself about calling so late: *This is a bad idea*, he thought. It was almost eleven o'clock, but before he could end the call, he heard Lisa's voice answer, "Hi, TJ!" In spite of the hour she sounded pleased to hear from him.

For a brief moment there was an awkward silence, but somehow TJ managed to get the words out. "Are you awake?"

"Yes, sure," she said surprisingly.

"Is it too late for company?" He let the ambiguity of that remark hang softly in the air.

"Of course not. Hurry up; I can't wait to see you!"

Not wanting to waste another minute, he motioned for Cameron to drop him off at his car.

"You're going to see her, aren't you?" Cameron asked.

"What makes you think that?"

"Because you're grinning like an idiot."

As soon as Cameron parked the Jeep, TJ opened the passenger door and jumped to the pavement below. Feeling as if the night was just starting, he waved good-bye to his friends and ran to his car. With a smile on his face, he drove toward Lisa's home on Sawmill Road.

Some four hours later, as a crescent moon lay suspended in the sky, he sat with Lisa on the couch talking and laughing about old times. He shared with her his goal of finishing nursing school in less than two years, and that he was more focused than ever to do something meaningful in his life to help others. Then his phone buzzed from a table nearby, the effervescence of the bell jar suddenly ending. Without even looking down at the name, TJ knew exactly who it was—his stepfather. After hearing Carey's concerned voice on the other end of the phone, TJ told him everything was okay, to go back to sleep, and that he was on his way. He grabbed his keys from the table and walked toward the door. As worried as he was about returning home to his parents, TJ was hesitant to open the door. He stood there looking at the pretty blonde on the couch and wished he could stay longer. All he could think about was when he could see her again.

"Maybe we can watch the Alabama game together this afternoon?" he asked, hoping Lisa would say yes.

"Sounds great! Just give me a call later."

He nodded and quietly closed the door behind him. Feeling like he was in a dream, TJ took in a deep breath of predawn air and walked to his car. As always, he strapped on his seatbelt before heading toward his parents' home some fifteen miles away. He glanced at the dashboard clock and hoped that his mom would be asleep. *She's going to kill me*, TJ thought, as he suddenly regretted not calling his mom and Carey to tell them he'd be out much later than midnight.

Some distance up the road, with his headlights shining brightly ahead, a sharp curve came into sight, so he slowed his speed and attempted to take the turn just as he had a few hours before. However, from the sudden jerk of his rear tires, he knew something was wrong—terribly wrong. Somehow, the car lost traction and began spinning and sliding out of control. He took a quick glance out the front window, but could only see his lights zigzag from one side of the road to the other.

He pumped the brakes hard, but there was no response. With the car spinning faster and faster, he feared that it was about to flip. TJ tried to jerk the wheel to the right, but he'd gone too far off the road to regain control. There were no shoulders or guardrails, making it impossible for him to stay out of the ditch. The tires made an awful sound, screeching on the blacktop and leaving a trail of skid marks behind. Holding the wheel with both hands, he steered more frantically, but nothing was working. The car was fishtailing and gaining momentum by the second. He thought: *This can't be happening*!

TJ felt a shock sprint through his body as he suddenly realized he was heading straight for a patch of sand. He looked up—the car was directly on course to a row of pine trees. If he didn't do something quickly, the car was going to hit the sand and fly into the trees. He jerked the wheel one last time, but it was too late. The car lost all traction, and he held tight to the wheel and braced himself for impact. The last thing TJ remembered before crashing into the forest was the headlights brightening the very tops of the trees like klieg lights illuminating a swaying sky. *This is it! I'm going to die!* Then in one powerful second, everything went black.

When he finally regained consciousness, TJ felt as though he was waking from a nightmare. Surely, this place must be Hell itself, and the devil's hiss now penetrated the still night. Just as his car was lodged between two trees, he could tell by the loud humming sound in his ears that the accelerator was stuck as well. Though TJ knew instinctively it was impossible for anyone to hear him over the whining engine, he clawed toward life. "Help! Is anyone out there? Help!" he screamed, waiting a few seconds before yelling again. "Help!" Yet again, no one answered. Looking blankly into the darkness, he had a terrifying feeling he was going to be there for a while.

The humming noise grew louder and louder, sounding as if the car was going to explode. With his fingers shaking nervously, he felt around for the ignition, but the steering wheel was ripped off the dashboard and the car's keys were nowhere to be found. Trying to think of a way to kill the engine, he forgot about the pain in his upper body. He turned his head from side to side, searching for a way out of the car. *I have to get out of here!* It was still dark, but he was able to see that each window had shattered and every surface of the dash was crushed.

TJ's first thought was not to panic, but instead to worry for his mom and other family members. *What will they do when they hear about this? I have to call Mom! She can't hear about this from anyone but me.* Still strapped into his seatbelt, TJ reached down to his pants pocket and felt for his phone—it was not there. With his hand down by his side, a strange realization crept over him. As his fingers moved across his legs, he felt no sensation.

"Oh my God!" he yelled, as he suddenly understood he could not feel anything from his chest down.

The breeze through the shattered windows felt much cooler now, and the row of pine trees before his eyes grew thicker. Never before had he dreamed just how completely he depended upon his legs. Never before had he imagined the world in which a paralyzed person lived. He had the sudden fear that his own ability to walk, to run and jump, to be in control of the simplest activity—of movement itself—was gone forever. His hips and legs were completely damaged. The thought brought a new burst of terror to his mind.

From an inch below his naval, his body felt heavy and swollen, as if a load of watermelons was stacked in his lap, cutting off all circulation from his brain to his lower extremities. As a nursing student at the University of South Alabama Nursing School in Mobile, he had learned enough to know this was serious. *Maybe my legs are asleep, or cramped from the impact of the accident.* He tried moving his toes, but because the dashboard and driver's side door pinned his legs to the seat, there was no way to check for movement. It was as if his feet were glued to the floorboard.

He also knew enough to reckon that the slightest mistake could damage his spine permanently, but TJ fought against panic and reached for the frame of the window anyway. He had to find a way out of the car, and from the loud humming sound in his ear, he knew the car was preparing to blow. As he lifted his arm, every breath required extraordinary effort, but he didn't give up. Feeling the chill of the early morning air on his forearm, he tried to reach the other arm across his chest but could not raise it above ninety degrees. From the deep pain in his shoulder, he realized his collarbone was broken.

Hopeless, TJ rested his arms in his lap and looked down at his hands. His pinky finger dangled off to the side, but this was by far not his greatest concern. He returned to the escalating noise of the V-6 engine, and to his fear of the car exploding with him inside. His heart raced faster and faster with each breath.

He rested his head on his seat and felt a cold sting at the back of his scalp, then rubbed his fingers through his blood-soaked hair. Tiny pieces of glass scraped against his palm.

This is bad. He knew now that if he had not strapped on his seatbelt before leaving Lisa's, his body would have been ripped into pieces and scattered through the forest like the leaves fallen from the trees.

Not able to do much else, he started to think about the severity of his injuries.

If I am cut and bleeding this much on the outside, he wondered, *how bad is it on the inside?*

He'd heard gruesome stories of people dying from punctured lungs, internal bleeding, and ruptured organs. If he were going to die, he didn't want to go without seeing his family again. *Please, someone find me!* He believed he couldn't hold on much longer—thirty minutes, maybe, if he was lucky.

Lucky. He'd always believed he'd been born on the sweet side of the day. But at this moment, he realized that luck shadowed every contingency, every plan, everything. Now, not only was he in excruciating pain, he was all alone and scared. He wondered about Lisa down the road. Would she be the one to find him like this? And what about the rest of his buddies? TJ had always been the strong one in the group—the one most of his friends depended on for help with their problems.

Again, he worried about his mom and stepdad. Carey had called to see where he was and if he was on his way home. TJ's mind raced. *How long had that been?* It was impossible to tell how long he had been unconscious, and the minutes now ticked by like drying concrete. Yet the darkness had not begun to thin to morning, and TJ knew that if they had stayed up to wait, his family was surely pacing the floors by now with concern.

Where is my phone? I have to call them.

He reached across the console and felt in the passenger seat. His cell was still nowhere to be found. He had no idea if his car was visible from the road, but he knew from the amount of blood on his hands and face there couldn't be much time left for him. His breath and strength were giving out. His awareness was dimming in waves of dizziness.

This could be the best sleep of my life, he thought several times, before a lecture from his clinical studies professor popped into his head. Suddenly he remembered his notes: *Trauma patients should remain awake and alert in order to avoid losing consciousness*, and, with that, a great rush of air slammed down his throat.

With the last remnants of his strength and will, TJ tugged on his seatbelt, trying again to free himself from beneath the dashboard, but he didn't get very far. His seatbelt was stuck; his legs were trapped; and the roof above his head had caved in too deeply for him to lift himself from the seat.

His frustration as acute as his fear, he thought again about his mom as he fought to stay awake. *How is she going to react seeing me like this?* he wondered. *She'll be upset and ask "Why now?" with everything going so perfectly in my life.* He thought of his nursing career and tonight's warm reunion with Lisa. He was finally growing up and making his own path. Everything was finally going right. *Why now?*

Glancing toward the sky, still a bowl of stars, he searched for answers. He didn't want to be a burden to anyone, especially his mom. He wanted to be strong and not have his family and friends worry about him. It was this realization, as much as the twinkling lights above, that drove him on. Then, as though a switch had been flipped, a sense of peace and understanding spread through his body. It was as if he knew everything was going to be okay. He would not die here.

All at once, TJ knew that in order to get through this, he had to pull himself together and acknowledge that he had been involved in a terrible accident, and that somehow it had been meant to happen. He closed his eyes and talked to the only other one there with him, "I'm so sorry, God, for everything I have ever done wrong. Please forgive my mistakes. I'm so stupid and I know that I've taken life for granted. Just let me live through this and I'll become a different person, I promise."

Suddenly, he saw headlights pass over, then come back—pausing—illuminating his car and the trees that held him in place. He strained his ears to listen for a voice, but the racing engine was too loud. TJ realized this was the most important plea he had ever made to God. *Help me now! Please let them see me.*

After waving his hand frantically through the broken window, trying to draw attention to being trapped in the car, he heard a loud voice. For the first time since the accident occurred, a tear streaked down his cheek. As he exhaled a deep sigh of relief, he knew this would not be his final plea.

"Help! I need your help to get out of the car!" He yelled as hard as his lungs would allow. In a daze of disbelief, and with the feeling of being the luckiest person alive, this time TJ heard what he had prayed for most: an answer.

1

IN SEARCH OF A CURE

Orange County, California
February 23, 2006

Two minutes before his alarm clock sounded, Hans Keirstead rolled over in bed and kissed his wife's shoulder. "Today is the day," he softly whispered, then eased from the covers, turned off the alarm, and began to dress, eager to get to his lab. For months journalists had stalked his every move, begging for the opportunity to interview him regarding his breakthrough—a treatment based on human embryonic stem cells that allowed paralyzed rats to walk again. This would become, arguably, the greatest scientific discovery since Jonas Salk invented the polio vaccine in 1954.

Of those journalists, Ed Bradley of *60 Minutes* had constantly been in touch with Hans, chronicling his accomplishments at UC-Irvine and reporting on the potential benefits of human embryonic stem cells. Bradley worked his contacts 24/7 and reached out to Hans on a weekly basis. He was fascinated by the science but was more impressed with the young scientist behind the research with whom he would be sitting down today.

Bradley, the tough, dogged reporter whose wide-ranging curiosity had taken him from the fall of Saigon to smoky jazz clubs and the sylvan halls of power, saw a huge difference in Hans from the other spinal cord researchers he'd followed. Most were much more logical, realistic, and methodical—they were okay with the slow drumbeat of scientific progress. Hans, though, didn't do anything slowly. He was not in the stem cell field to generate publications and write grants for more federal funding of research. He wanted to repair damaged spinal cords, and fast. Just as Thomas Edison had observed: Everything comes to the man who hustles while he waits. Edison might as well have been talking about Hans.

Born April 21, 1967, Hans Stegmann Keirstead was the fifth of six children. One of five boys, Hans understood at an early age that he would have to accomplish extraordinary things to rise out of the pack and make a mark. Watchful, hungry, and ambitious, it was easy for him to sit back and learn from his siblings' mistakes. And so, by example, he knew what he should and shouldn't do to make a good impression on the ones that mattered most—his mom and dad, Sandra and Kenneth.

His childhood was happy yet lean on a three-acre farm outside Toronto, Canada. The family of eight lived plentifully off the gardens they planted and the animals they raised. Hans's mother had been a local beauty widely regarded as both selfless and compassionate. His father, known as Ken to his friends, had come to Canada by way of South Africa, from a hardscrabble village known today as KwaZula, on the border of Mozambique. Born in 1940 to a family of missionaries, Ken learned the importance of helping those who were neglected, diseased, and impoverished, and vowed to instill the qualities of caring and humanity in his own family. Aspiring to do more for international health care of all people, Ken left Africa in 1957 to attend university and pursue a career in medical research.

Though Hans's parents divorced when he was in grade school, he remained extremely close to his father. It was Ken who taught by example and sparked his son's ambitions of medical school at a very young age. Hans would sit on the front steps of his parents' home and listen carefully as his father spoke about the importance of taking risks in life. Hans came to understand that failure was not falling down but staying down, and that strength could be gained by getting up. He learned that failure is double-edged, even acceptable, because that is how we learn. Failure drives achievement, and from that the young Hans knew that he would never set boundaries for himself, or be stopped by any barrier again.

At age eleven, after studying the central nervous system in science class, Hans decided that he wanted to work with that complex system of the body. He didn't understand the mechanics to it, or really what the central nervous system encompassed, but the idea of working with the brain and spinal cord fascinated him. The hope of developing cures for disease and injury took hold of his mind, crystallizing around a life in medicine. So, with a medical career in his future, Hans studied anything he could pertaining to drug therapy, rehabilitation, and clinical trials.

During his teenage years, he worked two part-time jobs to help his mother with expenses around their house and to save for college. If he was going to attend medical school, Hans knew eight years of college would cost much more than his parents could afford. After graduating high school in 1986, Hans emptied his savings account of three thousand dollars and began his undergraduate studies at the University of British Columbia (UBC). During his freshmen orientation, he learned that medical doctors applied existing knowledge, so in order to advance treatments for disease and injury, he decided to switch gears and earn a PhD instead of an MD. In other words, Hans didn't want to prescribe treatments, he wanted to *create* them.

In 1994, Hans completed his graduate degree and immediately began a postdoctoral fellowship at Cambridge University, England, his studies through university and graduate schools underwritten by grants from the Canadian government. It was during his neurobiology studies at CU that he realized there had been few discoveries in the field of regenerative medicine, so Hans, the thirsty child who wanted to achieve greatness, focused his research on the challenging work of stem cell therapy.

When he first started looking into creating a commercial and clinically viable population of cells, Hans knew human embryonic stem cells (hESC) could regenerate into virtually unlimited quantities and were the only cells that could make exact copies of themselves. But there were many social, legal, political, and ethical issues surrounding hESC technology. In the United States, where Hans had dreamed of being recruited after completing his postdoctoral studies, over three decades of public discourse and frustration had mounted over the use of human embryos for medical research.

Just the year before Hans's graduation from UBC, thousands of patients' rights and disease advocacy organizations spurred a movement which led President Bill Clinton to lift the 1974 congressional ban on funding embryonic stem cell research. This victory was short lived, however, lasting only until 1996 when Congress, in the form of the Dickey Wicker Amendment, banned yet again the use of federal tax dollars spent on research that creates, harms, or destroys human embryos.

Nevertheless, during this two-year window of support from President Clinton's administration, Hans witnessed huge advances in stem cell research. He became encouraged by the work of James Thomson and other American biologists who were being funded not by federal or NIH (National Institutes of Health) funds, but by philanthropists and biotechnology corporations around the globe. Hans was optimistic that if he could develop a proposal using hESCs and demonstrate a unique proof of concept, then he would have a great chance of securing private investors to fund his project through human clinical trials.

In the waning years of the Clinton administration, Hans delved into the laboratory and came up with an idea that had never been considered before, not even by Thomson who, in 1998, led the research team that successfully derived and cultured the first human embryonic stem cell lines. Hans did not envision implanting raw stem cells into patients because the cells might turn into undesirable types of tissues. His idea, instead, was to turn embryonic stem cells into the *desired* type of cell, such as cells that could specifically repair damaged spinal cords, in the laboratory and then transplant these more specialized cells into the patient.

Hans continued to develop his research, and in a matter of months had identified a novel concept for turning hESCs into a specific cell in the body, a process called cell differentiation. Hans felt his idea was a rare gem because many of his colleagues had spent years working to achieve proof of concept for cell differentiation—suggesting his idea had the potential for young cells to become specialized and take on individual characteristics to form a specific function—but none were close.

With his doctoral dissertation nearly completed, he began studying rats with spinal cord injuries because he had access to these animals at Cambridge and was able to conduct experiments easily. In the spinal cord, he would be able to tell if his stem cell therapy was effective simply by observing whether the animal's leg function improved; there would be simple outcome measurable effects.

The area of spinal cord injury, moreover, appealed to Hans because, although its effects are dramatic—compellingly so—it is nonetheless a one-time event, an acute injury sustained by immediate trauma to the spinal cord. He understood that had he focused on brain structure experiments, as many of his research colleagues were, he would have had to cut through the healthy tissues of a rat in order to get to the diseased or injured parts. Brain experiments did not interest Hans because it would have been impossible to get a rat to tell him how it was feeling, whether it had pain or had cognitive function. Hans wanted instead to make an immediate impact, so he made his decision as to where to concentrate his research based on a logical intellectual calculus that stem cell treatment might be the most effective therapy for spinal cord injury improvement. Now, with an amazing plan to manipulate stem cells into rebuilding damaged spinal cords, he started searching for financial support and a state-of-the-art laboratory to test his work and make things move quickly.

In late fall 1999, Hans accepted a position at the University of British Columbia's Collaboration on Repair Discoveries, a top Canadian spinal research center. This experience taught him quickly that in order for one to be successful in a career, one must be happy in the environment. His employer had been blunt: "It's going to be like this, kid. You work your ass off and I present your therapy as if it is my own, then in a few years you'll take my position and all the junior professors will work for you. That's how it works!"

Fielding his way at UBC, Hans was surprised to receive a call from Dr. Oswald (Os) Steward, the newly appointed director of the Reeve-Irvine Research Center in California, who invited him to UC-Irvine for a tour of the center. Hans was familiar with the RIRC, and admired its founders: the actor and stem cell advocate Christopher Reeve, and Joan Irvine Smith, a philanthropist and member of the family for whom Irvine was named.

During his visit, Dr. Steward said to Hans, "If I give you a sandbox to play in—and it's not going to be a fancy one—then I promise to take care of you and get you started, but if you fail, you fail on your own. You're not going to bring me or UCI down with you. However, if you reach the stars, then I am going to cheer for you, but I won't claim any of your success as my own. It will be all yours."

Dr. Steward's pitch attracted Hans immensely, not only for Irvine's healthy and sophisticated investment community, but because of the RIRC's research expertise and for other valuable resources he would need for his stem cell work.

Then, the deal-sealer: a phone call that very week from Christopher Reeve, the center's cofounder, who had become paralyzed after a horseback riding accident in 1995 and was today renowned as a national symbol for spinal cord injuries. Hans indeed respected the extraordinary Reeve more than any person in research and advocacy. As a champion for stem cell research, it was inspirational to watch Reeve influence public health care policy, as well as increase research dollars for stem cell research. And Hans wanted to be a part of this cause. He wanted to stand beside Reeve and help an entire community to one day walk again.

It was Reeve himself who personalized spinal cord injury for Hans. Reeve explained the struggles he encountered getting through each day—bladder and bowel control, sexual dysfunction, social stigmas—debilitating ailments that made life so much harder for him and other spinal cord injury patients. It was as if Reeve's drive came from some unknown force. Hans in turn would close his eyes at night and try to imagine what it must feel like to be told he could never be intimate with his partner or father a child of his own.

As Hans came to understand the crushing personal cost to those living with devastating spinal cord injury, he also came to realize the ripple effect this work would have on his own life. He recognized that he would be a terrible researcher with a broken heart. The stress and intensity of his work, the desire to mend lives, and the institutional and research barriers to surmount, were huge. So California, with its sunshine and curving hills, scalloped cliffs and indigo waters, seemed like a great place to call home. Moreover, the success, or failure, of his efforts, according to UC-Irvine's Dr. Steward, would be his alone.

Just as Christopher Reeve believed, Hans knew that human embryonic stem cells were magical and could become *every* cell in the human body. But there lay the young scientist's greatest challenge: how to coax stem cells to become only *one* cell type—the spinal cord cell type lost after spinal cord injury. And, how could he generate pure populations of spinal cord cells, free from contaminants, such that they could be used in human clinical trials?

With many believing these challenges to be unsolvable, Hans devised a plan to speed up the bench work by hiring skilled scientists, and to expedite the FDA approval process by recruiting experienced regulatory officers. Hans refused to be another scientist who discovered something amazing, only to get left behind without the means to manufacture it or apply it to medicine. Reeve believed in Hans, and so did Os Steward. Hans felt it was the perfect time, and the RIRC the perfect place, to put his plan in motion. He signed on.

2

PROTOCOL

Reeve-Irvine Research Center
Irvine, California
2000–2006

Preparing for his meeting that day with Ed Bradley, Hans's mind floated back six years to where his professional career began in the United States. In 2000, just two years after Thomson's isolation of hESCs, Hans joined UC-Irvine as an assistant professor and saw his name mortared onto the wall of the Keirstead Laboratory at the Reeve-Irvine Research Center. He was just thirty-three years old.

Written into his contract with UC-Irvine was that the Keirstead Laboratory would remain at nonproductive status for one year in order to recruit skilled staff, install computers, move in equipment and microscopes, and hire regulatory officers who would keep track of upcoming experiments. While establishing his training programs for preclinical studies, Hans was cautious of the political, funding, and scientific environment, and chose his resources wisely.

On August 9, 2001, President George W. Bush placed restrictions on federal funding for embryonic stem cell research. In a national address announcing his decision, watched by millions of Americans, Bush stated that federal funds could only support research using human embryonic stem cell lines created before 9 p.m. that evening. At the time of the announcement, it appeared that there were roughly seventy lines available for federal funding, but further investigation reduced that number to twenty-two lines, and many of those older lines were showing signs of mutation and other problems after so many years of growing in a lab.

Regardless of these challenges, Hans was optimistic about his protocol and pushed forward to find quality samples of his primary source of research—human embryonic stem cells. As he contemplated the use of federal and nonfederal stem cell lines, Hans decided to sidestep the Bush administration, with their ongoing political maneuvering and conflicting policies on stem cell research. Hans felt this was much too big of a hassle to use dual laboratory space and equipment for working with federal and nonfederal stem cell lines, so he looked to the highly sought after H1, H7, and H9 lines discovered by James Thomson back in 1998.

Hans knew from his years at Cambridge that Geron Corporation in Menlo Park, California, had funded Thomson's research and had negotiated the intellectual property rights to his invention—endlessly dividing cultures of hESCs—which could address the deadliest diseases and injuries on the planet, including cancer, heart disease, diabetes, and spinal cord injury. Using every possible resource, Hans called up a former college girlfriend who now worked for Geron and asked for her help in getting those stem cells.

Just three weeks after President Bush announced his restrictions on federal funding for hESC research, Hans attended a meeting at Geron, bringing with him his PhD dissertation on spinal cord regeneration, in order to show these stem cell experts he had found a way to restore spinal cord function in paralyzed rats. Thomas Okarma, Geron's CEO, was impressed, and a few weeks later, Hans returned, this time to further explain his idea to senior management about the nuts and bolts of his proposed stem cell treatment. Hans suggested that if Geron provided the stem cells for his research, he would make the world's first high purity population of any stem cell type.

The decision was easy for Geron: working with Hans Keirstead was a perfect fit for the 180-person biotech firm. The company's goal was to develop cell types from human embryonic stem cells that had potential therapeutic applications as cell therapies to address chronic and degenerative conditions. And this was exactly what Hans brought to the table.

In cooperation with the young scientist, Geron ended up sponsoring Hans and his laboratory at UC-Irvine, giving him $500,000 per year for as many years as it took to bring the therapy to human clinical trials. This was a critical moment for Hans. The partnership immediately made him an invaluable asset for the university and reinforced exactly what his father Ken had emphasized years before: in the world of biotech engineering, such partnerships were as inevitable as they were essential. An academic lab, no matter how well equipped or financed, could only go so far without private support and funding. Hans and Geron merged together and formed a phenomenal team; it was one in which Hans exceeded their expectations—and they his, by providing financial security, academic direction and support for his spinal cord injury research.

Finally came the breakthrough Hans had dreamed about. It was a tireless and frustrating process for the Keirstead Lab, but in 2002, their hard work and persistence paid off. Hans and his team were able to prove they had discovered a high purity population of oligodendrocytes—a tricky word for an important cell in the nervous system that supports neurons. Neurons are nerve cells, the cells (or wires) that carry messages from our brains to our spinal cords. These particular cells make an important protein called myelin. The oligodendrocyte cells wrap themselves around neurons and the myelin serves as insulation, much like that in electrical wire.

Inside the Keirstead Lab, the spinal cord of a rat was exposed surgically and then bruised with a blow from a small, blunt object to simulate spinal cord injury in humans. After the injury, the animal was unable to use its hind legs. It could move them a bit because the injury was not complete, just as is the case sometimes in humans. But the animal was dragging its belly, an indication that there was no consistent coordination between its front and hind paws.

After a spinal cord injury, many neurons—the cells carrying the information from our brain to our body—are lost forever. Others simply lose their insulating cells (aka oligodendrocytes). When this happens those wires can no longer conduct electricity, or signals from the brain, resulting in paralysis. But Hans's breakthrough came when he took cells from the H1 line and influenced them to become human oligodendrocytes that make myelin to protect those signals. When he transplanted them into the rat's injured spinal cord, it restored the function of the neurons that were still alive but had lost their insulation as a result of the injury. In the case of the rat, it was enough to restore the animal's ability to walk again.

In a video that Hans shared with national media, the rat named Fighter, who previously supported her weight with her belly off the table, now displayed locomotion with coordinated front to back movement of her front and hind paws, and her tail was up—which indicated an amazing degree of recovery.

Hans's news stunned research laboratories across America and invariably divided the research community into two groups—believers and skeptics. Some scientists respected the young neurobiologist but hesitated to believe that a treatment for spinal cord injury could be found in this microscopic cell called an oligodendrocyte, and Hans's approach had never been attempted before, so there were no results that could be confirmed or papers published to support his unique approach. Still other scientists argued that the risk of tumor development from these cells was too high. That fear alone was enough to make most experts reluctant to jump on board.

Nevertheless, Hans and Geron pressed forward with the research and decided to take their therapy to the next level: human clinical trials. Hans didn't want to treat rats for the rest of his life; he wanted to treat humans, but in order to move forward with human clinical trials, he had to help Geron replicate his oligodendrocytes in large mass production. After all, humans are larger in size than rodents, so for treatment purposes there had to be a bulk supply of these cells, millions upon millions of them, in fact.

Hans had developed a forty-two-day procedure during which stem cells were exposed to many different combinations of growth factors and hormones—the longest differentiation program in existence, and the only one in the world to make a high purity population derived from stem cells. So he knew his process: Hans knew he needed oligodendrocytes to produce myelin, and he knew that to provide enough of these cells to do any good, he would need mass volumes of human embryonic stem cells. Now, he had to figure out where to get them from.

Obtaining the cells from cadavers or fetal tissue wouldn't work, as these cells would be of different developmental stages and contaminated with other cell types. Furthermore, one could just not get enough cells from these sources to treat the thousands of new spinal cord–injured patients each year. Although other stem cell types were available, their yields were simply too small for commercial success and none replicated themselves as well as embryonic stem cells.

After seeking advice from a college friend at the NIH, Hans learned that over 500,000 blastocysts (the hollow ball of cells that forms a few days after an egg cell is fertilized, also known as an embryo) that had originated in petri dishes were stored at fertility clinics across North America. Moreover, 10,000 of these blastocysts were being destroyed each week because of time constraints or financial burdens to the couples who could not afford the expense of keeping these blastocysts frozen in liquid nitrogen tanks, or had given up hope of becoming pregnant altogether. If frozen for longer than ten years, these blastocysts became nonviable tissues and, therefore, could not be donated to other couples. So, for these reasons, Hans went after these abandoned blastocysts as his primary source for treatment and cure.

Unlike religious and social conservatives, who would rally otherwise, Hans did not see an immediate moral or ethical dilemma in using these abandoned blastocysts for research. In fact, he valued these cells just as much as any human rights group or religious group in the country would. He, too, felt that they were sacred cells, and he couldn't fathom the idea of tossing them into a dumpster or damning them to a freezer for eternity. He believed, furthermore, that there was no clear right or wrong answer to this moral dilemma; but, as the marine biologist Rachel Carson once observed, "The materials of science are the materials of life itself." Somehow, Hans was going to have to try to address that impenetrable dilemma as best he could.

His team wasted no time in obtaining the consent of couples with embryonic tissue that was destined to be destroyed. From these blastocysts, he extracted human embryonic stem cells—the cells that are capable of becoming every cell in the human body. These were the cells that he used to make high purity populations of oligodendrocytes that were identical, easily expanded, and human.

Just five years after joining UC-Irvine, Hans published his airtight research in the *Journal of Neuroscience* on May 11, 2005, reporting that he and his team had carefully coaxed these cells into oligodendrocyte progenitor cells (OPCs) and had successfully injected them into rats with acute spinal cord injuries. Most impressively, six weeks later, these rats could walk again.

Hans's findings may have taken three years to publish, but he gave due diligence to testing and retesting his process, making certain that everything was perfect so when he stamped his signature of approval on the publication, the study would be 100 percent accurate and proof of concept well established. Indeed, Hans's findings proved that these animals could bear weight on their hind legs and move their tails from side to side. Even reluctant scientists took notice that these rats demonstrated improved motor function below the level of injury—a first in any stem cell clinical trial. It was a degree of recovery that had never been achieved in any clinical study before.

And so, for these reasons, Ed Bradley had purposefully chosen Hans for the *60 Minutes* piece on stem cell research: this scientist who, unlike so many before him, was young and charismatic—he could relate to the audience and engage them with this controversial topic better than anyone else in the world.

Hans was just as compelled to speak to Bradley, someone who shared his passion for treating spinal cord injuries with humanity. Hans wanted the country to move forward with supporting stem cell research and finally put to rest the outrageous and entirely false claims of killing babies for science.

As the broadcast began, in an effort to defend the ethical manner in which his research was conducted, Hans explained that he and his team were not destroying lives, and certainly not farming women's eggs. As the interview with Bradley proceeded, the handsome thirty-eight-year-old neuroscientist explained the concrete benefits of stem cell therapy to one of America's favorite and most trusted journalists. But even this veteran reporter had not anticipated the outpouring of interest that came during the three-minute interview, when human embryonic stem cell research was removed from the secretive walls of research labs, universities, and technology investment firms and entered the homes of millions of ordinary people.

In a relaxed, easy-to-understand manner, Hans explained that the human embryonic stem cells used in his studies were not derived from aborted fetuses—that is, a blastocyst that successfully implanted inside a woman's uterus and began to develop into a fetus (which generally occurs after eight weeks of development), then was terminated either by an induced abortion or ended spontaneously from natural causes. Instead, Hans's cells came from an abandoned blastocyst that had been frozen at a reproductive center. Hans made it clear that he did not create these blastocysts, but instead was granted the cluster of cells after couples donated them to medical research or had abandoned them at fertility clinics.

With his hand balled into a fist, he compared the casing of the blastocyst to that of a tennis ball: the outer layer, the one that you "see," he explained, controlled the destiny of the approximately 150 inner stem cells. But, he continued, if the outer layer of the tennis ball was removed, basically, the instruction manual for the inner stem cells was removed as well. That is, it was no longer recognizable as a tennis ball and could really become any ball whatsoever. In other words, these inner stem cells could be manipulated to become any other type of cell, growing their own new covering. They could become the base cell for any part of the human body—in the instance of his research interest, the casing for new spinal stem cells. Hans, apparently, had proven that the impossible was, in fact, very possible. He made it sound easy—elementary even—but the six-year road to get to that point had been anything but simple.

Because of Hans's disarming hunger for a cure, sudden interest in stem cell research became widespread. In homes, schools, and churches, seemingly overnight, just like Hans had hoped, people were finally paying attention. But with the good came the bad. With Hans's results now public, the viability of usable stem cell therapy began to become more realistic, and thus those in opposition to stem cell research became ever more vocal against it. Many feared this would ignite a firestorm of new concerns among antiabortion and pro-life groups across America.

However, a week after the *60 Minutes* interview aired on February 23, 2006, over 380,000 letters addressed to Hans Keirstead flooded the CBS News mailroom in New York. The letters covered a range of topics and issues, but the majority clearly applauded this medical breakthrough as stem cell therapy tapped into the hopes of millions of Americans—who now could finally believe that a cure for disease and injury might actually happen in their lifetime.

It's true that Hans's stem cell success would not have been possible without the teamwork and commitment of the Keirstead Lab. In the stack of papers being prepared by Geron for submission to the FDA, Hans saw the lives of dedicated and loving human beings and the millions of patients and medical doctors at rehabilitation centers across the globe. The harshness of a disability and the elusive search for an answer renewed Hans's determination day after day, driving and guiding him to spend nearly every waking hour in the lab.

3

FROM BENCH TO BEDSIDE

California
2002–2009

With Hans back in his laboratory at UC-Irvine and working on other targets for stem cell therapy, a team of people at Geron took his stem cell protocol and began to manufacture a large-scale "industrialized" production of Hans's cells for clinical trial and commercial use. This was by no means a simple process and required many phases: Have you ever noticed how you can cook something very successfully for two or even five people, but when you try to make the same dish for a dinner party of twelve or twenty, suddenly it just doesn't work out the same way, or taste as nice?

The same problem occurs when going from a small culture dish of cells in a research lab to the many and much larger cell culture flasks that are required to generate a much larger number of cells. This kind of challenge was well known in the biotech industry as something that had to be worked through, whether a company was manufacturing a protein, an antibody, or a cell. In this case, making mass quantities of stem cells was extremely complicated, and even more so when working with human embryonic stem cells.

Adapting the protocol so that all of the reagents and ingredients used were suitable for clinical use in humans was a hugely expensive process for Geron, with over $1.8 million being pumped into the initial research for the kick-start of the trial. Developing a manufacturing process to generate Geron's treatment, known as GRNOPC1, to current Good Manufacturing Practices (cGMP) was another necessary step, and still undefined in many ways. Good Manufacturing Practice is an internationally recognized and accepted system that ensures errors do not occur during product development. For the Geron trial, it was crucial that its stem cells be consistently produced and controlled according to quality standards. A successful outcome would help boost global pharmaceutical opportunities for the new stem cell therapy.

During the final weeks of 2007, Geron scientists finalized all of the "release tests" that the manufactured lots of GRNOPC1 were subjected to before being turned over for use in preclinical safety and efficacy studies, and then in the clinical trial itself. The scientists also collaborated with engineers to develop a syringe-positioning device for injecting the cells into the damaged spinal cord of the patients, and created a training regimen for the surgeons to follow during the injection procedure. After years of consulting with expert neurosurgeons and engineers, Geron scientists had developed the protocol for their stem cell clinical trial.

Because Geron was eager to move their spinal cord program into human studies, the company worked around the clock to prepare supporting documents for the U.S. Food and Drug Administration. The FDA, through its approval process, makes the final call as to whether the benefits of a drug's use outweigh the drug's harms. The FDA also helps to ensure that the drug's labeling adequately warns doctors and patients of the known risks.

In 2008, after spending $20 million for preclinical development, Geron felt confident they had met the criteria to persuade the FDA to allow the first federally regulated clinical trial using human embryonic stem cells. This Phase 1 trial would not aim to cure patients but to establish that the cells were safe to use in humans.

Since 1997, the FDA has required registration of clinical trials to be made through the National Institutes of Health (NIH) in order for the federal agency to monitor and measure the outcomes of each phase. In summary, there are four phases of a clinical trial. Phase 1 typically includes 0–100 patients who are tested to determine if the drug or treatment is safe for humans (causes no harm); Phase 2 includes 100–300 patients who are tested to determine if the drug or treatment has any efficacy (may work); a Phase 3 clinical trial includes 1,000–3,000 patients in order to determine if the drug or treatment has any therapeutic effects (it works); and Phase 4, which is not required by the FDA, includes anyone seeking treatment with the already approved drug or new therapy from their physician. These patients are then monitored for long-term effects.

In multiple rounds that resulted in over 22,000 pages of research and data, Geron submitted its application to the FDA in March 2008. The review process lingered on though, and before the FDA could rubber stamp the trial, Geron discovered that the rats being treated with GRNOPC1 had begun to develop skin-like cells growing on the spinal cord where they shouldn't. These nonproliferative (they do not grow) cysts were harmless masses, like microscopic water balloons, but they did not belong at the injury site. As a precaution, Geron asked the FDA to put their application on hold so they could perform additional research and prove that these issues had been resolved.

Back in the laboratory at UC-Irvine, news of Geron's willingness to report their negative findings did not surprise Hans Keirstead, but it did impress him. Geron was not legally required to report this information. But Hans had worked with Geron scientists for many years, and he knew the level of integrity these experts exercised. He felt it was admirable for a company to imperil their own product and investment for transparency, and for the truth. Certainly an honorable decision to make, but it did lengthen the application process.

For another year then, Geron scientists adjusted the manufacturing process in order to prove their treatment was safe to test in humans. GRNOPC1 produced by this enhanced recipe was injected into more than a hundred rats and subjected to extensive toxicology testing to support its IND (investigational new drug) application and thus begin human clinical trials.

The United States had made vast improvements of the process since the modern clinical trial was born in Britain during 1948. It was during this time of repair after World War II that a study of streptomycin for the treatment of tuberculosis was conducted. This was important because tuberculosis had been the most important cause of death in young adults in Europe and North America. This study was also a first to control variables by both randomizing the patients to different study arms and blinding (masking) the arms so that neither patients nor researchers knew who received which treatment until the study was completed. This design, referred to as a randomized controlled trial (RCT), became the gold standard in medical research and was intended to produce results that were verifiable and statistically significant.

And so once again Geron was prepared to take Hans Keirstead's spinal cord treatment from the bench to the bedside—meaning they needed the FDA approval *and* human patients to enroll in the clinical trial. On January 23, 2009, just three days after President Barack Obama's presidential inauguration, a media explosion occurred with news that FDA approved the application for the Geron trial to begin. The story was carried by almost every news source around the globe.

Some thought the approval of the first hESC trial was due to the new president's support for federally funded research during his campaign. Obama would officially declare his position two months later by overturning the Bush administration's ban on federal support for hESC research. On March 9, 2009, President Obama issued an executive order to fund "responsible, scientifically worthy human stem cell research to the extent permitted by law."

Under these new guidelines, stem cell lines would need to be derived, with the proper informed consent from the donor, from leftover blastocysts (embryos) that fertility clinics would have otherwise thrown away. Obama's new policy had immediate impact, with nearly two hundred human embryonic stem cell lines becoming available to NIH-funded researchers.

Indeed, the approval of the Geron trial was a turning point—a landmark—when public and scientific excitement was at an all-time high. Many felt the perseverance of Hans and Geron demonstrated the potential of stem cell breakthroughs and helped pull the United States out of the political quagmires that had held back the advances of science and medicine.

4

WHISPERS TO HEAVEN

Chatom, Alabama
September 25, 2010

Saturday morning came too soon for Caleb Fights as he stepped outside his dad's home on Sawmill Road to start the 6 a.m. shift at the local grocery store in Chatom. The sixteen-year-old didn't mind working the weekend shift; it was the six hours of stocking shelves that he disliked. He would rather work the register or sweep the floors any day of the week rather than bend and straighten over a thousand times during any one day.

Before the screen door slammed behind him, he heard a whining sound that echoed through the dense layer of pines surrounding his dad's property. The trees leaned in to each other so closely, it reminded him of a family, like a protective hug. But in this morning's stillness, Caleb listened carefully and was certain that what he heard wasn't the sound of an animal. It sounded more like a revved engine, and he wondered if a couple of the local boys had been out racing and that perhaps something had gone very wrong. He was dressed and ready for work, so he jumped into his pickup and sped to the end of his driveway. With his headlights shining across Sawmill Road and into the forest, he immediately spotted a red vehicle wrapped around a pine tree with its front tires spinning out of control. Instead of panicking, Caleb parked his truck and scanned the area for other vehicles or bystanders.

Unable to see much through his own dark and dusty windshield, he opened his door and poked his head out into the cool morning air. Caleb was terrified to go near the roaring car. It sounded as if it could explode at any moment. *There is no way that anyone could survive that*, a thought that passed through his mind as he eased back into the driver's side seat of his pickup. But something pushed inside his stomach and urged him to take a closer look at the car.

Although it was still dark, from the glow of his headlights it looked as if someone had taken a four-ton Coke can and crushed it between two trees. Caleb wanted nothing more than to put his truck into reverse and start his daybreak commute all over again; however, he knew that wasn't an option.

Unfortunately, he had now entered into TJ's nightmare.

Parked twenty feet away from the wreckage, Caleb could only make out that all four windows had busted, and that the car had crashed into the forest tail-end first. He sank back into his seat and hoped the morning sunlight would reveal the accident was not as bad as it appeared.

If anyone is in the car, Caleb thought, *they're gonna need help to get out.* He was terrified of seeing someone dead in the car. It had only been a year since he and his father had come across a scene just as horrific as this. Suddenly the memories of that tragic accident came rushing back to him. Caleb closed his eyes and could see the bloody baseball cap and tennis shoes splayed across the road, a gruesome bread crumb trail leading fire and rescue volunteers toward the body.

Unfortunately, the teenage driver of that vehicle was thrown so far into the woods that it took several canines to find his remains. Caleb hoped the driver of this vehicle had not suffered the same fate. He looked up and prayed that somehow he or she had found a way to safety.

Caleb drew a deep breath and opened his truck door. Stretched on the tips of his toes, he could barely see the dash of the car; it had shifted to the right passenger seat along with the frame of the windshield and the roof. With the car sounding more and more sinister, like a snarling metal predator, he thought it was best to return home and wake his stepmother.

As the headlights tapered away through the pines, TJ's cry for help went unanswered yet again; his shallow voice was no match compared to that of the roaring engine. *Oh God*, he thought to himself, *I'm going to die out here alone!* He was near the point of giving up. Hopelessness was setting in, and he was a tangle of bone, blood loss, and misery; but again, he thought of his family and focused on staying alive.

Slowly, he tried to raise himself by pulling on the seatbelt strap, but the frame of his car had shifted in a ninety-degree angle, which made it difficult to grasp the strap. The pain from his broken collarbone was becoming more intense, and his good arm was too weak to stretch across his upper body. It seemed as if everything that could go wrong had. His only hope was that the wrinkled morning sunlight would allow a passing driver to finally see his vehicle in the woods. *Surely someone will find me*, he thought. But with no watch or dashboard clock or cell phone to tell him how long he had been there, he worried that his body could not hold out long enough to be rescued.

Even though he was covered in blood from head to toe and feeling no sensation below his waist, TJ didn't lose faith that God would get him through this. He had never been angry with God before, and this was not going to be the first time to be so. Instead, he was angry with himself for taking everything for granted: his family, friends, and independence. *I've been selfish, stupid, and careless*, he thought. In that moment, he realized that he had been given every opportunity in his twenty-one years of life and had wasted so much of himself on unimportant things. Even so, he had always had a gift for looking life square in the eye. At that moment, lying flat on his back, he knew his injury was more serious than a pinched nerve or a swollen disk. There was still hope, though fading against the red thread of a rising sun. If he survived this, he knew the use of his legs might be taken away forever.

Staring at the break of light above, he only wished he could turn back the hands of time and be an independent person again—free to walk and run, to go and do as he pleased.

Returning to prayer, he closed his eyes and whispered toward the heavens above, "Dear Lord, please let me live. I promise if you see me through this, I will never go back to living the way I did before this accident. Please, Lord! I'm begging you to send someone to find me so they can call Mom. I just need to hear her voice."

Dust trailed behind Caleb's pickup as he rushed home to wake his stepmom, but Nichole was already up and running her bathwater in the back of the home. She had just turned off the faucet when she heard a loud commotion outside her bathroom door. It only took a few seconds to throw on her robe and make her way down the hallway into the kitchen. Immediately, she knew something was wrong by the sickly gray expression on Caleb's face. He was standing near the kitchen table, raking his fingers through his hair. "What's going on?" she asked, hoping all it was was something he had forgotten for work.

"Oh God!" Caleb shouted. He was trembling all over and could not get the words out fast enough. "You've got to get to the end of our driveway. Someone has wrapped their car around a tree."

It was the terrified tone in his voice that convinced her to open the door and listen for herself. Immediately, the sound of the engine in the distance caused Nichole to step into her husband's sneakers and run to the back of the home to wake her nine-year-old daughter. There was no landline phone in their home to call for help, so Nichole would have to use her cell phone which she hoped was somewhere in her car. Without another passing second, Nichole ran to the carport door with her daughter K'leigh following closely behind. She instructed Caleb to drive to her sister's home and wake her from bed. "I don't care what excuse she gives, Caleb. I need you to meet me at the end of the road with Debbie as soon as you can."

Nichole didn't want her young daughter to be alone in the car, especially not knowing if there might be any fatalities at the scene. With Debbie living just three miles down the road, she was the closest person to keep an eye on K'leigh.

Not a minute later, Nichole parked her car at the end of the driveway and shined her headlights across the road. It was impossible to miss the red metal wrapped around the tree. Being from a small town, she feared whose daughter or son, husband or wife it was who had crashed into the forest. She pushed away her panic, gripping the steering wheel so tightly that three of her acrylic nails popped off and shot into the floorboard near K'leigh's feet. Her heart felt as if it was going to burst from her chest. She had never seen anything like this before and could not imagine how anyone could survive.

Glancing over at her daughter, Nichole could tell by the shaking silhouette in the window that K'leigh was a nervous wreck from the terrible sight. Instead of jumping out to see if there were any victims, Nichole felt it was best to stay put with K'leigh and call for help until her sister arrived. "Where is the phone, sweetheart?" Nichole asked and felt around in the darkness for her BlackBerry.

K'leigh was in a state of shock and did not respond.

Unsure if her daughter was distracted by the noise or traumatized by the scene before her, Nichole took one hand from the steering wheel and nudged her daughter's leg. "Baby, are you okay?"

K'leigh's chest was heaving up and down and tears poured down her cheeks. She didn't understand why this had to happen at the end of her driveway at six o'clock in the morning.

In a firm voice Nichole said, "K'leigh! You have to snap out of this and help me find my phone. We need to call 9-1-1."

Nichole tried to remain calm for them both, but the engine was only getting louder. She flipped on the interior light and felt around in the console for her phone. After throwing her checkbook and Ray-Ban case on the floorboard, she saw the hot pink cover and snatched it up.

"Lord, please help us!" she shouted after realizing the battery was dead. More frustrated than ever, she popped the glove compartment open, grabbed the cell phone charger, and instructed K'leigh to connect it to the cigarette lighter. With the cable connected and battery signal blinking across the screen, Nichole knew it would take a few minutes before it was charged, so she opened her door and ordered K'leigh to stay inside the vehicle.

"Honey, I'm going to step outside for just a minute to see if anyone is in the car. You stay put."

K'leigh turned her head and nodded, but she didn't say a word. She was no doubt afraid, but she understood that someone could be trapped in the car and in need of their help. She was very content to stay inside the vehicle.

Nichole had never been trained for a serious rescue situation like this, but fortunately her work as a medical receptionist had given her the confidence and determination needed to take control of the situation. She had seen every case imaginable, from a man who entered the office with a pair of scissors stuck in his chest to a woman who delivered a baby in the waiting area. She had experienced her share of blood and gore.

Just as she reached for the door handle, she saw a bloody arm wave across the beam of light and then drop to the side of the car. She grabbed K'leigh's leg and squeezed tightly. "Did you see that?" she asked nervously. "There's somebody in the car. Oh my goodness, they're alive."

K'leigh shrank back in horror against the passenger side door and the tears began to pour once gain. Nichole hated to leave her daughter so upset, but she knew the person in the car needed her help more. She reached for the handle again, gave a quick pull, and then jumped to the ground below. She sprinted across the sandy path toward TJ's car. Just steps away from the wreckage, she could smell gasoline but didn't turn back. This made her realize she was putting her own life at risk, but the waving hand only encouraged her to run faster to the car. Nichole had no idea that she was about to become one of the most important people in TJ Atchison's life. She was only seconds away from becoming one of many heroes that day.

The car was on a muddy bluff, and wedged so tightly between two trees that the front tires were off the ground and spinning at over twenty miles per hour. Nichole moved quickly up the hill, screaming each step of the way. "Hello, can anyone hear me?"

She saw the hand move again, so she screamed louder. "I'm almost there. Can you hear me?"

She made it to the driver's side of the car and followed the bloody arm to a shadow in the seat. The engine was still blaring, so Nichole leaned into the space and screamed as loud she could, "Are you okay in there?"

There was just enough light from the headlights to help her determine there was only one person in the car. It was a boy, a very young boy. She heard his voice, it was weak, but she was relieved to hear anything at all.

"No ma'am," he answered, "I can't feel my legs and my collarbone is broken."

His words sent chills down her spine. No wonder he could not get out of the car. But once again, she thought it was a miracle he had even survived this.

Whatever emotions stirred inside her head, she focused on TJ's face and was amazed by the calmness she found in this young man's eyes. Her own eyes strained to hold the terror within. She had no idea how severe his injuries were, but guessing by the missing steering wheel and imploded dashboard, she knew he needed immediate medical attention.

"Are you in pain?" Nichole asked, hoping he could not feel the console crushing his legs. Her goal was to put his mind at ease. "My name is Nichole Fights, and I live just up the road." She pointed toward the driveway just two hundred yards away. "I'm here to help you!"

TJ exhaled deeply. He was not okay, but he felt much better knowing she was there and he was no longer alone. "I'm worried about my legs. I think my back is broken."

"No, baby. Everything is going to be okay." Nichole said in calm voice. "What's your name?"

TJ stammered, "My name is TJ Atchison; I'm twenty-one years old and in nursing school. My parents are Timmy Atchison and Anita McDonald."

"Okay, TJ. I know your momma. She kept my son at her daycare when he was little. Do you know her phone number so I can call her?"

"No ma'am!" he said. "Please don't call her just yet. I'm afraid she is going to be upset with me for wrecking the car."

As a mother herself, Nichole knew his mother would be relieved to know her son was alive. However, she didn't want to upset TJ. "Okay, baby. I'm going to stay with you and hold your hand until help arrives. I think you're going to be fine, but you've got to have some help to get out of the car." This was a far cry from the truth. Nichole knew TJ was in big trouble, and if help didn't arrive soon, things could take a turn for the worse—for them both. The car, she feared, was a ticking time bomb. But she was not going to leave him.

Out of the corner of her eye, she saw the headlights from her car flicker on and off. Still holding TJ's hand, she rose to her feet and saw K'leigh hanging out of the driver's side door waving her cell phone high in the air.

Nichole gripped TJ's hand tightly and said, "I'm going back to my car to call for help. I won't be gone long, but it's too loud to call from here."

"Please don't leave me," he begged.

"I have to do this, TJ!" It was hard for her to leave him, but she knew he wouldn't make it much longer with the amount of blood he was losing from his head. "I promise, I will only be gone for one minute."

She gently placed his hand on his chest and gave a reassuring smile. "I'm going to try and turn off the car, but if I can't reach the keys, we're gonna have to think of something else to stop the engine." She stretched her arm across the driver's side seat and felt for the ignition, but the entire dash was out of place and caved in too deep to reach anything. She wasn't giving up hope that she could somehow stop the engine, but for the moment, it was more important to call 9-1-1 and get help on the way.

The bright digits on her phone read 6:12 a.m., and the battery signal was at two bars. She had just enough juice to make the call. From then on out, every second counted.

5

CLEARED TO LAUNCH

Orange County, California
July 30, 2010

It was a slow morning for Michelle Goldman, the twenty-six-year-old assistant at Reeve-Irvine Research Center in southern California. She sat in her six-by-six cubicle and surfed the Internet, hoping to find something of interest in the day's science headlines. It took only seconds for her eyes to lock in on the company's name she'd heard a hundred times in the last year: *Geron to Proceed with First Human Clinical Trial of Embryonic Stem Cell Based Therapy.*

Michelle leaned in closer to the screen and read the first lines of the press release to make certain it was related to the same clinical trial her boss had worked on for over eight years. There it was, confirmation, in the final words in the paragraph—six letters ending with the number one, GRNOPC1—that gave notice her day was going to be anything but ordinary. This was the news she and Hans Keirstead had been waiting on for weeks since getting a call from Geron to be on the lookout for an announcement "any day" from the FDA. Finally, the green light had been given for their spinal cord therapy to be tested in a human clinical trial.

Michelle jumped to her feet—her checklist for the morning was quickly thrown out the window. Her immediate objective was to find Hans and tell him the exciting news. Standing on the tips of her toes, she could barely see over the five-foot partition that separated her desk from the dozen other workspaces in the laboratory.

Other than the mice in their cages and a maintenance supervisor who could outwork any young intern on campus, the large, stark space looked abandoned. Michelle's calf muscles began to cramp and a lump formed in her throat. The thought occurred that she had somehow overlooked an internal email about the FDA granting Geron Corporation permission to move forward with the trial. What if everyone was downstairs celebrating right now? She was almost in tears. She hated to be the last to know about anything—especially about an issue involving her boss and the Reeve-Irvine Research Center.

The petite blonde snatched her bag from the chair and raced toward the door. With each passing step, the feeling of déjà vu grew stronger. She, Hans, and the rest of the staff at UCI had been down this road twice before, because Geron had run into regulatory snags in 2008–2009 that had delayed the trial until now. However, this time something felt different. With a new, pro–stem cell administration in Washington supporting the research, she felt certain the clinical trial would proceed.

Suddenly, the doors swung open and a tall, handsome man appeared with a cup of coffee in one hand and the other holding a data report. The forty-three-year-old who looked more like a gleaming movie star than a stem cell pioneer nodded good morning and then continued briskly past her without saying a word.

She followed the smell of hazelnut Dolce DaVinci and watched him closely. Nothing seemed unusual about his demeanor today. Hans was always in a hurry, as though time was a fast-moving river that could not carry in a day a fraction of what his brain wished it to.

Surely he knows by now, Michelle thought, but as Hans made his way down the hallway, she knew by his composed demeanor that he had not yet heard the big news. She watched only a second longer before she called out, "Hans, you know about the FDA approval, right?"

His brisk pace came to a sudden halt. "Approval of our trial?" he turned and asked with a look of disbelief across his face.

Michelle took a deep breath. *He has no idea.*

"Yes, I just read the announcement online. It looks pretty solid, Hans. I hope you are ready to celebrate?"

Still ten feet away from her, he put the data folder under his arm and reached into his back pocket for his wallet. A second later, he walked toward her holding a wad of cash. A huge smile crossed his face. "No,

Michelle. Today, we are going to celebrate for millions of people." His eyes brimmed with tears as he put the money in her hand and asked, "Do you have time for a quick errand?"

Overjoyed with excitement, she answered, "Anything for you, boss!"

At 10 a.m., Michelle returned to the center with a case of Veuve Clicquot in the backseat of her charcoal gray 2009 BMW 328i. She paged Maintenance and asked for someone to send a cart around to help her unload the bottles.

Once inside, the maintenance supervisor followed behind in a near sprint, trying his best to keep up with the young assistant. Michelle pushed the cart onto the elevator and managed to catch her breath before the doors opened on the second floor. She heard the sound of cheering and excitement echoing down the hallway as they wasted no time in wheeling the cart into the laboratory filled with scientists, administrators, interns, and dignitaries from the community. Michelle began passing bottles of Veuve Clicquot around the room.

Standing near a table of microscopes, Hans's eyes sparkled more than ever as corks shot across the laboratory and champagne began spilling over onto the floors. Glasses were filled and arms raised as toasts were quickly made. It was a time for cheering and celebration, a culmination of a lot of hard work and dedication from every person in the room, with dozens more celebrating four hundred miles away at Geron headquarters.

I only wish Christopher were here to see it—then it would be perfect, Hans thought, as he remembered the actor and stem cell advocate, who had become Hans's close friend before passing away in 2004 from complications of spinal cord injury. Wiping a trail of tears from his cheek, Hans embraced the moment with his colleagues and wondered if the same emotions he was experiencing now were also felt by the scientist Jonas Salk back in 1955, when his polio vaccine was approved by FDA.

Feeling humbled before the accomplishment of this team, Hans expressed his gratitude to the UCI staff and administrators who shared in today's achievement. It was in fact so dreamlike that Hans needed to see the FDA announcement for himself to make certain it was real. He walked over to an empty cubicle and scrolled the cursor across the computer screen. He held his breath as the words he had worked, waited, and prayed for for nearly a decade appeared—*First Human Clinical Trial.*

July 30, 2010. The date affirmed that what some skeptics had called insane and idealistic science was not so crazy after all. For millions of doctors, nurses, injured, sick, and suffering people and their loved ones—for the world at large—this day created hope for stem cell cures.

6

A RACE AGAINST TIME

Chatom and Mobile, Alabama; Atlanta, Georgia
September 2010

Fire Chief Benjamin "Ben" Jones of the Chatom Fire Department received a page from 9-1-1 dispatch at 6:13 a.m. on Saturday, September 25, 2010. The code read, *1050 vehicle located on Sawmill Road,* which told him that an automobile accident had occurred and passengers were trapped inside.

In less than six minutes, Ben, his brother Benyan, and volunteer fireman Ron Lonergan were strapped inside the fire truck and en route to the scene.

The adamant, breaking daylight revealed itself to the crew as they turned right onto County Road 1 and drove six miles west toward Sawmill Road. Regardless how much training the three men had, nothing could have prepared them for what they were about to see.

Just fourteen minutes after receiving code 1050, Ben turned a sharp curve and saw red flashing lights straight ahead. With the engine roaring and his fire siren blaring, he punched the gas pedal and sped down the open stretch of road.

He scanned the area quickly and saw a red car crushed between two pine trees. It looked as if the car had flipped in the air, hit a tree and then fell to the ground only to become wedged between the two trees.

The crew wasted no time as they grabbed as much gear and equipment as they could carry and sprinted across the sandy ground. Benjamin's immediate responsibility was to access the vehicle to determine how best to rescue survivors inside. His first question as he passed a paramedic, "Is anyone alive in there?"

The paramedic said, "Yes, there's a driver alive and responding."

Based on the condition of the car—the entire frame was beaten and bowed upward on both ends, all windows busted out, and the driver's side door frame shifted over the driver's head—Benjamin understood it was a race against time to save him. He knew there were sophisticated tools inside the fire truck, including new burst hose, valves, and extraction tools and that his team was well trained in their use, but in this particular instance the wreckage resembled a crushed child's toy. The slick brown needles of the pine forest were covered with twisted metal and glass crunched beneath his boot. Ben knew that in this deep morning stillness it would be a miracle if the driver survived.

With the car facing south, Ben approached the passenger side and glanced in to see a paramedic starting an IV on a bloody hand. He scanned the driver's face but didn't recognize TJ at all.

The paramedic was doing everything possible for him, but there was absolutely nothing more she could do but remain calm and wait until the door frame was removed above TJ's shoulders.

A two-foot post ran from the top of the windshield down to the dash, pushing his left leg into the floorboard. A fallen tree had pinned TJ's leg very tight, making it extremely difficult for Ben and his team to extract him. Ben realized instantly the only way to get TJ out of the car was to cut him out using the Jaws of Life.

With a loud siren approaching from the distance, Ben was relieved to see Laton Hill Fire Department pulling in next to his truck. Now, he had two sets of everything, including two Jaws of Life and several other volunteer firemen to help peel off the roof of TJ's car.

The Chatom crew started snapping posts behind the driver's side door using a Sawzall to cut the tinier pieces pinning TJ's leg. TJ talked to Ben the entire time, telling him about his nursing classes, asking lots of questions about his car, his legs, and wanting to know if any family or friends had made it to the scene. "I'm sure they are here," Ben answered but never took his eyes off TJ's face.

Ben had no idea that TJ's father, Timmy, was speaking with a paramedic near the tree line, begging for information about his son.

Even though the car was a mess, Ben was most concerned about TJ's legs, and wondered why the young man could not feel the steering wheel shaft piercing into his right knee. Hoping it was just a pinched nerve, he asked, "Hey, TJ, can you move your legs out of the floorboard?"

"No, Sir! I can't feel anything below my waist," he answered.

The paramedics stepped away from the car to allow Ben, Benyan, and Ron plenty of room to maneuver the large hydraulic scissors in and out of the door frame and around the hood. Using every muscle in their bodies, they finally were making progress cutting through the metal. Thirty minutes later, the roof was slowly pulled away from the car and thrown to the ground.

Ben turned toward the fire trucks and saw a crowd gathering in the distance. It was extremely helpful for his crew that no one, including TJ's mother Anita and stepfather Carey, had attempted to interfere with their rescue efforts. In his twenty-seven years as a first responder, this was the first time that bystanders had not tried to take matters into their own hands by moving debris from the scene or trying to help the injured involved in the accident.

Now that it was bare and exposed, Ben saw that the inside of the car was completely demolished. The dashboard and console had shifted to the passenger side, along with parts of the steering wheel and airbag, which had not deployed.

Exhausted from his injuries and weakened by extensive blood loss, TJ complained of being tired and wanting to go to sleep. Ben and the paramedics knew they had to extricate him before he became unconscious, so they placed a C-collar around his neck and called for a backboard. Ben, Benyan, Ron, Ralph Morris, and Steve Burton positioned themselves inside the car to extract TJ from the driver's seat and transfer him to the backboard.

With Ben lying across the center of the car facing TJ, he reached through the busted windshield and deep into the floorboard to grab hold of TJ's ankles. In a firm voice, Ben began the countdown, "THREE - TWO - ONE - LIFT!"

At the same time, LifeFlight air transport hovered above the wreckage, searching for a clear path to land. With a level spot in sight, the

LifeFlight pilot lowered his chopper, causing a mighty sand-storm. Quick to react, Ben and his crew used a nearby tarp to cover TJ and protect his wounds from the stinging sand and debris.

Knowing that TJ was minutes away from being airlifted, Anita ran to the female paramedic who had cared for her son during the extraction and asked where he was being transported.

"USA Medical Center," the young woman answered.

Anita pulled her husband's arm and motioned for him to follow her to their car. She was determined to make it to University of South Alabama Medical Center, some sixty miles away in Mobile, before Life-Flight landed with TJ.

An hour later, he was admitted into the emergency room at University of South Alabama and surrounded by dozens of family members and friends who had been rushed to Mobile in a police-escorted convoy. Doctors treated TJ's immediate wounds—right clavicle fracture, left fifth finger dislocation, facial lacerations—and then performed an MRI, which confirmed their preliminary diagnosis of paralysis. TJ had experienced a burst fracture at thoracic level seven of his spinal cord and would need surgery to stabilize his spine.

Surgery was performed two days later on September 27, 2010.

After meeting with his surgeons and learning that TJ was completely paralyzed from the chest down, Anita took the elevator down three levels to the hospital waiting area so that she could quietly process the upsetting news. With tears streaking down her cheeks, memories of her son's very active twenty-one years drifted in and out of her mind.

She was angry at God, then her frustrations shifted to TJ for staying out so late. She even blamed herself for not getting to TJ and the wreckage sooner. With her hands shaking by her side, Anita took a deep breath and realized there was no one to blame for her son's accident—not God, not TJ, and not herself. She knew life would go on regardless of whether her son could walk or not. TJ was strong and would adjust, and they all would. They would help each other. TJ was alive, and that was all that mattered.

After a while, Anita composed herself and stood up. She returned to the elevator and searched for a quiet place to make a call. She was going to have to break the devastating news to her father. He and TJ had always been exceptionally close. She would have to remain strong for her parents and the other family members, all of whom were in shock and tears.

Just as the elevator doors were about to close, a young man in a wheelchair stuck his hand inside. Anita watched him push himself inside the elevator. He appeared to be the same age as TJ, and from his calm expression, she guessed he had been in a chair for some time. Looking at the curl of dark hair against the boy's neck, she saw her son. Trying her best to contain her emotions, Anita was unable to hold back the warm tears that filled her eyes. As if time stood still, she envisioned TJ trying to go about his daily life in a wheelchair. It was a thought she could not imagine.

Anita swallowed hard and realized this moment that had brought the two alone together in the elevator was no coincidence. As the doors shut, she tapped the young man on the shoulder and in a soft whisper asked what led to his paralysis. He turned his head and gave her an unexpectedly warm smile, as though he too recognized the urgency of the moment. He'd been involved in a car accident, he explained, paralyzed from the chest down for over five years. She was surprised to hear him say that he was changed for the better, and appreciated life, family, and his friends more than ever before his accident.

The young man listened as Anita explained that her son had a very similar diagnosis. He detected the sadness in her eyes, so he did his best to calm her fears by stating that the doctors said he would never walk again either. And yet now, after four years of aggressive rehabilitation, he could stand and walk with assistance. He looked at Anita, his eyes clear and alive. "Tell your son not to give up! Miracles happen every day," he told her, and in that moment she made a promise to remain hopeful and optimistic that TJ would indeed walk again.

When the elevator doors opened on the third floor, Anita ran toward her husband and family with a new outlook on her son's diagnosis. This encounter motivated her to find TJ the best rehabilitation center in the United States. On the top of her list was Atlanta's Shepherd Center, recommended by a family friend, Bonnie Blackwell, who had also suffered a spinal cord injury several years before. What Anita did not know was that Shepherd, along with Northwestern University Hospital in Chicago, had recently been approved as the first two sites selected to enroll patients in Geron's stem cell clinical trial, with seven other locations to be announced soon. While neither rehab center was yet authorized to recruit patients to the clinical trial, inquiries from patients could be made to begin the qualification process.

On Wednesday, September 29, 2010, four days after the accident, Anita dialed 1-800-SHEPHERD and was connected to an admissions liaison. Just a few minutes into the conversation, she was asked all types of specific questions about TJ's age, his health background, the level of his injury, and more. As Anita responded to each question, she was curious why the liaison on the other end of the phone was so excited and eager to schedule TJ for transport to the rehab center. Before she could learn more, Anita's cell phone dropped the call and she was unable to dial back until the following day.

In the meantime, Anita downloaded and completed the admission forms from Shepherd's website. Still unaware that Shepherd was participating in a historic clinical trial, or that her son met the inclusion criteria that would make him the first patient injected with human embryonic stem cells, Anita faxed in TJ's insurance information, family medical background, consent forms, and a routine but nonbinding letter of intent for TJ to participate in any of Shepherd's clinical research studies if he met the criteria.

As the fax came through at Shepherd, it was as if an alarm sounded, with dozens of staff members scrambling around the rehab center to notify top administrators that a potential transplant candidate was soon heading to Shepherd.

TJ was called first thing Friday morning, October 1, with news from the Shepherd Center to pack his bags and be ready for air transport that afternoon to Atlanta, Georgia. The clock was now ticking for TJ to be enrolled as the first candidate in Geron's human embryonic stem cell clinical trial.

By 4 p.m. (EST), TJ had settled into his room at Shepherd, with his mother, stepfather, and grandfather one block over, unpacking their things at the Family Center. An hour later, a team of doctors entered his room and asked if he would consider participating in a research study. Thinking all rehab patients were somehow involved in research therapy at Shepherd, TJ said, "Sure," and then agreed to read through the protocol.

He was handed a twenty-page document and scanned the cover page.

Protocol: #CP35A007

INFORMED CONSENT AND AUTHORIZATION TO USE AND DISCLOSE MEDICAL INFORMATION; A PHASE 1 SAFETY STUDY OF

GRNOPC1 IN PATIENTS WITH NEUROLOGICALLY COMPLETE, SUBACUTE, SPINAL CORD INJURY

Sponsor: Geron Corporation 230 Constitution Drive

Menlo Park, CA 94025

Investigator: David F. Apple, M.D.

1. Purpose and Background

You are being asked to participate in this research study because you had a spinal cord injury within the last 7–11 days. The main purpose of this research study is to assess the safety of GRNOPC1, an experimental cell-based agent.

GRONPC1 is not approved by the US Food and Drug Administration (FDA). GRNOPC1 is made by Geron Corporation.

Your study doctor is being paid by Geron Corporation to conduct this study.

GRNOPC1 contains a mixture of cells that are made from human embryonic stem cells. Most of the cells in GRNOPC1 are a specific type called oligodendrocyte progenitor cells. Laboratory studies have shown that the cells in GRNOPC1 promote partial repair of the damaged spinal cord tissue in animals with a spinal cord injury. These studies also showed that GRNOPC1 promoted partial improvement in the ability of some animals to move their back legs. GRNOPC1 has not been given to human subjects prior to this study, so it is not known if GRNOPC1 will give any benefit to humans with spinal cord injuries.

This study will see if it is safe to inject GRNOPC1 into a person's spinal cord between 7 and 14 days after their injury. This study will also assess the safety of GRNOPC1 for 1 year after it is injected.

A total of 8–10 subjects who are between the ages of 18 and 65 years of age will take part in this study. After a subject receives an injection of GRNOPC1, no more subjects can begin participation in this study during the next 30 days. The study will be conducted at multiple centers in the United States. Your participation in this study will last for about 1 year.

If you agree to participate in this study, you will be asked to take part in a long term followup study. You must agree to take part in the long term followup study in order to participate in this study. This is required because

> the long term safety of GRNOPC1 is not known and the cells cannot be removed from you after they are injected.
>
> Long term followup is also required because the original human embryonic stem cells from which GRNOPC1 is made were grown on a layer of mouse cells. More information about the human embryonic stem cells is provided in the next section of this consent form. The long term followup study will be explained in a separate consent form. Your participation in that study will last for 14 years after you finish this study (15 years total).

TJ raised the back of his bed and looked up at the doctors and at his family now entering the room. He was surprised the protocol mentioned stem cell therapy. He'd heard about stem cells in nursing school, ironically just two weeks before his accident. He was aware of success stories using stem cell treatments for bone marrow transplants and felt optimistic this brand-new, untested protocol could be his best chance to get better. The document left him intrigued and hopeful that a potential treatment was available, and that he could be the person who helped make stem cell research a reality for others.

Over these last turbulent days, TJ had tried hard to focus on gratitude and not on what he had lost. Regret, he had intuitively come to conclude, was a terrible waste of energy. You can't build on regret, but you can build on ruins, and that was what he had to do now. To build a new life for himself, accepting that meant he would never walk again, or maybe, just maybe he might. *What do I have to lose?* he thought.

He asked the doctors to leave the room so he and his family could discuss the pros and cons of his participation in private. He knew he wanted to become part of this, but recognized that the treatment was not without controversy. That much he knew about human embryonic stem cells. He wanted his family's thoughts, and most important, their approval.

Thirty minutes later, TJ's door opened and Anita walked out into the hallway to retrieve the research team.

With a heart full of hope and a confident stroke of his pen, TJ signed the consent forms and handed them to Dr. David Apple, emeritus medical director of the Shepherd Center and principal investigator (PI) for the Geron trial. It was Dr. Apple's job to make certain everything ran smoothly at Shepherd. Most importantly, as PI, Dr. Apple was in charge of making sure the protocol was followed precisely by his colleagues and staff.

Dr. Apple took the signed protocol and placed it inside a folder marked CONFIDENTIAL. It was quiet in the room as the research team and family members contemplated the significance of what lay ahead. A few seconds later, TJ managed his first smile that day and said, “This is my only shot, the closest thing I can do to ever walk again. I’m in!”

And the tests and procedures began.

7

THE TRIAL BEGINS

Atlanta, Georgia
October 2010

A major challenge for Geron was that participants in the study had to receive their GRNOPC1 within fourteen days of the injury. This crunch period was required because of secondary injuries—scarring and inflammation—that spread like wildfire around two weeks after the initial injury. This scar tissue prevented the stem cell treatment from reaching the damaged nerves. Just as the body rushes to form a scar around the injury site, so too must the newly injured patient hurriedly decide whether or not to participate in the trial.

As soon as TJ was admitted to Shepherd, the study team had to quickly initiate the process of assessing his vital signs, performing physical exams, electrocardiograms, and MRI monitoring. Blood samples were collected to test for HIV, hepatitis B and C, and for evidence of any other serious diseases or infections that might impede TJ's ability to participate in the trial and in the follow-up evaluations.

The study team was relieved to see that all tests came back negative. TJ's immune system looked stronger than ever. Dr. Apple was optimistic that TJ would remain healthy and be able to receive the stem cell injection as scheduled for October 8.

TJ was still firmly committed to the trial and to moving forward with the procedure, but his deep spiritual roots were telling him to reach out to someone in the ministry. Specifically, he wanted the counsel of the pastor whose services he'd attended several times that summer, Brother Troy Bailey of Reynolds Holiness Church, and he wanted his prayers. TJ picked up his phone and called him.

Back in Chatom, Troy Bailey listened intently to TJ on the other end of the phone. He could hear the nervousness in the boy's voice and could only imagine how overwhelming this decision to participate in the trial had been for TJ. Immediately, Bailey said yes. He packed an overnight bag and made the seven-hour trip to Shepherd Center to pray with TJ before his life-changing surgery.

On October 7, with TJ's family gathered around his hospital room, Brother Bailey sat at the edge of the bed and listened as TJ explained his position about embryonic stem cell research. With his eyes wide and confident, TJ said, "This surgery is not taking a life. It's not like these cells are coming from an aborted fetus or anything like that. They're going to be thrown away in a garbage can."

Just a few minutes into the conversation, TJ learned that his pastor adamantly opposed stem cell research, as did thousands of others from back home who were pro-life supporters. However, Brother Bailey believed this experimental treatment was acceptable because the cells had been obtained from embryos that would never be implanted in a woman's womb, and so they had no chance of developing into a baby. Everyone in the room was in opposition to abortion or the use of fetal cell tissue in research.

But not everybody back home, or in the pro-life movement generally, understood the nuances involved in this particular treatment. And so in a heartfelt and concerned voice, Bailey asked, "Are you aware that millions outside of this room are going to look at this procedure and disapprove of your participation? There will be opposition against you, TJ. Many will not share your views on human embryonic stem cell research. Some may even make threats against you. Are you prepared for this?"

"I believe everything happens for a reason, and my gut is telling me to do this," TJ answered.

"I understand, TJ. However, the publicity you receive may not be positive!"

Anita spoke up and said, "Even if it's bad, this will make TJ and our family stronger. God is our leader and we are putting this in His hands.

If TJ makes it through surgery okay, then this is what was meant to happen all along."

TJ did not waver either. His decision was made, and he was ready to proceed with surgery. Brother Bailey reached across TJ's bed, grabbed his and Anita's hands, and led the family in prayer. He thanked God for the blessings of that day and asked for strength and wisdom for what was to come.

When Dr. Donald Leslie jumped in his car Friday morning, October 8, 2010, he felt honored for the role he was about to play on this historic day. Dr. Leslie, a Shepherd spine surgeon and rehabilitation specialist for over twenty-seven years, was at the top of his medical career as medical director of Shepherd and coinvestigator of the Geron trial. But regardless of the number of surgeries he'd performed or the accolades attached to his name, assisting Dr. Apple with this important protocol was by far the most incredible experience of his medical career.

Just a few weeks before TJ was admitted to Shepherd, the same study team had screened and approved another patient (Patient X) for the Geron trials. Only hours from surgery, the young man had decided not to participate as the result of being spooked by an article he read online. Patient X feared the stem cells implanted into his spine would grow body parts or organs from his back.

Dr. Leslie explained as best he could that none of the animals in the laboratory had grown ears or kidneys in their spines, and Geron did not anticipate this would happen in humans. Nonetheless, Dr. Leslie respected his patient's concerns and knew that coercion was illegal, unethical, and a malicious way to advance science. And after all, the cells being used in the Geron trial were a foreign substance that had never been injected into a human before. This was the main reason why the safety trial was so important to Dr. Leslie and the Geron team. The single goal of this Phase 1 trial for the enrolled patients was to prove these cells did no harm when injected into the human body. Patients had to do a risk assessment and decide whether they were all in or not.

It had been a tedious and disappointing process. Four other previous candidates had made it to surgery day, and each had been disqualified for one or more of these issues, often associated with spinal cord injury: spiked fever, acute infection, blood clot, blood pressure issues, bowel problems, and/or respiratory problems. Dr. Leslie and his team, therefore, were hopeful yet cautious this morning, too, that TJ develop neither complications nor second thoughts about his participation. The team ardently believed, due to his age and "can-do-it" attitude, he was the perfect candidate for the Geron trial.

Dr. Leslie arrived at Shepherd Center before dawn. The rest of the medical team was already there: Dr. Roger Frankel, the young neurosurgeon from Piedmont Hospital who had been trained by the Geron team to perform the injection; Dr. David Apple, Shepherd's principal investigator for the trial; Dr. Edward Wirth, Geron's medical director; one anesthesiologist, two nurses, and the engineer who designed the syringe-positioning device. For the patient's sake, Dr. Wirth, along with all the other participating spine surgeons, had spent over a year rehearsing the complicated procedure, practicing it under different scenarios, so they could be ready for anything and act quickly.

Because the injection of GRNOPC1 had to be exact, Geron designed a positioning tool that attached to the frame of the operating room table and enabled the spine surgeon to precisely control the needle placement and penetration into the lesion site. Dr. Frankel and the other participating spine surgeons were trained six months leading up to the surgery in the use of this device as part of the clinical trial site initiation protocol.

At 7 a.m. the group walked directly across the street to adjoining Piedmont Hospital. The syringe device and surgical equipment had been housed at Piedmont in a special operating room, with two sets of everything in case something went wrong with the first set.

Once inside the operating room, doctors Leslie, Wirth, and Frankel examined TJ's MRI images one last time before surgery. They wanted to position him under the device so that the cells could be injected approximately five millimeters below the center of his injury. Wirth recommended this for safety reasons because he didn't want to take a chance on the injection damaging the intact tissue above the injury; but at the same time, he wanted the cells to be close enough to the center of the injury in hopes they would spread throughout the injured area and repair the damaged nerves. In military terms, it was a little like lining up a bombsight over a target.

Wirth had handpicked the radiologist who would analyze the images from a remote location and forward them to Geron headquarters. Wirth studied the images closely to make recommendations on the injection site, but the final decision would be left up to Dr. Frankel. The group's assessment was, however, in sync with one another, which was very encouraging to Wirth. The nervous tension among the group was palpable, and yet they were ready. The injection site was identified. The OR team was in place to connect the attachment piece to the operating table. And TJ had already been transported to Piedmont an hour before, prepped, and given medication to help make him comfortable and relaxed.

There was an awkward moment for the medical team when he was rolled into the operating room, because they were not supposed to identify their patients. The group did their best to respect TJ's privacy and to not interact at all with him. At the same time, they wanted him to know how much they appreciated his commitment to the research, so they lowered their heads as he entered as a show of respect.

Considering the circumstances, TJ was very calm and ready for the surgery to begin. Wirth positioned himself next to Frankel to make certain every step went according to the protocol. With a nod from Frankel, the anesthesiologist shot a clear medication into TJ's IV to make him unconscious. As soon as they had him under anesthesia, Frankel inserted a long needle into TJ's lower back and performed a lumbar puncture to retrieve spinal fluid, which would be used as a baseline for comparative monitoring in the weeks and months ahead.

With TJ on his hospital bed and turned on his side, Frankel withdrew the spinal fluid needle and the surgical assistants transferred TJ onto the operating table. Dr. Leslie stepped over to the table and helped Dr. Frankel cut the incision down TJ's back.

Once the engineer had the positioning device set up, Wirth took an empty syringe and needle and mounted it into the frame. He and Frankel slowly moved the frame over the location they wanted for the injection. They lowered their magnifying scopes and turned on their headlamps. Everything was in place.

In the meantime, the oligodendrocyte progenitor cells had already been delivered from the transport facility some twenty miles away. The cells were delivered to the operating room perfectly on schedule. With the empty syringe in one hand, Frankel removed the fluid-filled syringe from the cooler with the other and held tight as Wirth connected a sterile needle. The duo performed several steps to get the cells primed into the needle, and then Frankel loaded it into the positioning device. Then he carefully maneuvered the needle to exactly where he wanted it at the spinal cord.

After movement and pulsation was noticed on TJ's exposed spinal column, Frankel asked the anesthesiologist to turn off the ventilator so his young patient would lie completely still for the injection. That's when things became a little tense for the team, because now the clock started ticking for TJ to be off oxygen. The maximum ideal time for a patient to be off a ventilator is between five to ten minutes because after that, their blood oxygen levels can start dropping and carbon dioxide can start building up, which is dangerously problematic.

So once the ventilator was turned off, everything moved quickly. Frankel and Wirth got the needle down to the spinal column and a tiny incision was made into the area, then through the muscle, and then finally pierced through the bone to expose TJ's damaged spinal cord.

The room was silent as the device slowly lowered to a half-inch above TJ's spine. The tension was palpable because everyone knew the procedure from here on had to go exactly as planned. A nurse behind Dr. Frankel started calling out ten second intervals on the clock.

With a push of a button, the needle went smoothly in, and Frankel completed the injection in under two minutes. This was followed by a two minute hold time to allow the two million cells just delivered into TJ's spinal cord to disperse around the injury site before Frankel withdrew the needle. These extra minutes prevented any cells from leaking out of the area. With two minutes allotted to withdraw the needle, the anesthesiologist kept a close eye on the clock. A total of six minutes was all they had for the entire injection procedure. Frankel's timing had been perfect, but he also needed to make certain his technique had been perfect as well. Taking a deep breath, he leaned over TJ's spine and exhaled an enormous sigh of relief when he saw that no fluid had leaked out, nor had the injection caused any bleeding.

With TJ back on the ventilator, Dr. Frankel and Dr. Leslie closed up his back, deeply gratified that the surgery had gone well. Their hands had done the preparation and closing, and the device had injected the magic cells. Now it was up to TJ's body and the cells to determine if human embryonic stem cells would be found safe for human therapy.

8

HEAD IN THE CLOUDS

Millry, Alabama
September–November 2010

In late September of 2009, I went out on a limb and created an outline for a story that had been brewing inside my head for months. For an hour, as the sun burned the sky to copper, I sat on the back porch of my family home and filled ten pages of what would eventually become a 100,000-word manuscript.

With graduate school during the day, and the tests and assignments that would advance my degree in elementary education, I researched and wrote during the small hours of the night. It was exhausting, no doubt, and terrifying, too. "I am a writer who came of a sheltered life," Eudora Welty once explained, though sheltered life could be a daring one too, for "all serious daring starts from within." I thought she might as well have been describing me. Either I allowed my imagination to roam freely, or chained it down and suffered through the consequences. I chose to go where my thoughts allowed and braced myself for the ride.

Four months later, after pouring my heart and soul into the tremendous effort, I was thrilled to have finished my first young adult novel. My goal for the new year was to find a literary agent who believed in the story and would want to represent me. In the meantime, I had four wonderful children to look after, whom I hoped would one day be proud, or forgiving, of the passion that held and exhausted me as I eased out of bed at midnight to finish one chapter and awoke before daylight to begin a new one. I was in this to learn and grow as a person, but also to help others, including my kids, discover their own passions of life. I knew this adventure might not result in anything monetarily, and that was completely okay. I had found something greater inside that had challenged me like never before. For these reasons, I would endure the ups and downs that would come my way.

During the next few months, I kept writing, and sending out submission letters. I jogged to release the stress and tension and learned to embrace the exquisite lessons of patience. In March 2010, I created a blog called Head in the Clouds where I documented my writing experience.

An optimistic attitude, I knew, would be crucial to my success. Shortly after connecting through my blog with other writers, I learned the query process could take anywhere from a few months to even years. This seemed unbearable to my family and friends, but after enduring two years of fertility treatments and months of bed rest with two of my pregnancies, and then losing my second daughter to preterm delivery, I had already grown resilient toward heartache and uncertainty. As the polite decline letters from agents trickled in, I learned quickly to let rejection roll off my shoulders, and focused on the positive responses I had received. And to my surprise, there were four literary agents who liked my query letter and requested to review the complete manuscript.

Full of enthusiasm and excitement, I couldn't wait to share the wonderful news with those I loved most. My parents, the best proofreaders in the world, shared in my time of joy. But my husband of ten years, the one person I wanted to please more than anyone, had lost interest in me and our marriage. Several months into 2010, I noticed him slipping away from our children and me, both emotionally and physically. His work and diversions were of greater joy to him than spending time with our family. Determined to save our marriage, I reached out to our pastor to schedule sessions for marriage counseling. Time and again, my husband failed to show.

And so feeling bewildered and broken, I had to find an outlet, a way to release the frustration and sadness. My therapy became writing and exercising, which drastically improved my page output each day and helped me shed those last thirty pounds of pregnancy weight.

Then one afternoon, I experienced sharp pains in my lower back while barely making it home from a long run. I knew intuitively that something was terribly wrong with my body. I called my mother, and she drove me to the local infirmary where an ultrasound revealed large, grape-like cysts on both kidneys. The technician asked if there was a history of kidney disease in our family. Tears filled my eyes as I remembered my Aunt Toby, who suffered through three years of dialysis before she died in November 2007 from complications of polycystic kidney disease (PKD).

And now, I had PKD, too, which meant that if the law of averages held, two of my four precious children would likely be diagnosed with it in their lifetimes if a cure were not discovered. Worried for all of us, I started researching online for everything I could find about kidney disease. I learned that PKD causes clusters of fluid-filled cysts to grow on kidneys, which could eventually lead to kidney failure. But my greatest concern was reading that PKD could also affect the brain or heart. If PKD affects the brain, it can cause an aneurysm—a bulging blood vessel that can burst, resulting in a stroke or even death. My parents, siblings, and closest friends were kind and encouraging during this difficult time. But the person I needed most, my husband, was not there to hold my hand and support me. I would have to deal with the diagnosis without him.

In August, just days before my twins, the middle of our four children, began kindergarten, I realized my marriage was dangling by a thread. The children's father packed a suitcase large enough for a month's vacation and walked out of our home. Still asleep inside, my little miracles had no idea our family would forever change.

A month later, feeling exhausted and discouraged, I received an email from a top literary agent offering to represent my young adult novel if a few minor revisions could be made before the holidays. Dreading the idea of the word "revision," I replied: "Absolutely! I'll make the recommended changes and return the manuscript before November 1."

There were no second guesses or fears of rejection. I had to come through for my kids, so I rolled up my sleeves and went to work.

Considering the mayhem at home, the first week of revisions went extremely well. Fall was in the air and my spirits were improving daily. I was feeling positive and good about myself for the first time in a long while and completed nearly half of the edits in less than ten days. Then I came home on a beautiful late Sunday afternoon to find my husband standing on our front steps. In a low voice, his head down to avoid eye contact, he said he wanted to give us another shot.

I was hesitant to trust him, or to allow him back into our home, but our youngest three children, who, hearing their father's voice, had come to the door, seemed so happy to see him back home again. That first evening, as he slept on the couch downstairs, I got on my knees in our bedroom and prayed that time would heal the sadness and disappointment still bottled up inside.

A week later, on the eve of my thirty-third birthday, my parents agreed to babysit the children so my husband and I could spend some time together, away from work, chores, and our unhappy relationship.

The trip gave us time to rest and begin to repair, but I knew by my husband's silence and blank stare through the windshield on the drive home that he was miserable and wanted out. The next day he was gone again, and this time for good.

TJ's accident occurred the following Saturday, and even though my entire life had turned upside down, I regrouped and shifted my attention to helping my best friend and her son.

TJ's mother Anita and I had been friends for nearly ten years. We met when she began babysitting my nephews, and then several years later my own children started trickling through her day-care center. Anita became like a sister to me. She knew everything there was to know about me and vice versa. We shared personal hurts and pains of life and often picked one other up when times got too tough to bear.

When my mother called very early on the morning of TJ's accident to tell me he'd suffered a severe injury to his spinal cord and was at that moment being taken by air ambulance to a regional hospital, I could only imagine the terror and dread gripping this family I had known and loved for so long, as though they had all been pulled into the inner circle of hell.

Anita and I exchanged Facebook and text messages, but I waited until two days after TJ's surgery at University of South Alabama before visiting his family. My three-year-old daughter Courtney and I made the trip to Mobile, arriving just before noon on September 29. We brought candies and cards from my other children, along with a gift card for Anita to help with the incidentals she incurred while away from home.

With Courtney in my arms, I walked off the elevator and found Anita and her father sitting in the family waiting area. Dozens of strangers circulated the room, but we stood frozen in time, stunned by TJ's devastating paralysis. I wrapped my arms around my friend and told her I would help in any way she needed.

When I went in to see TJ, the impact of the trauma he had experienced was far greater than what I'd expected to see. And yet despite the gashes and stitches, and the bandages and sling from a severe clavicle fracture and, of course, his very still body, his sweet smile radiated throughout the room. I leaned over TJ's bed and gave him a soft hug, wishing a miracle would happen and his body would heal completely. For half an hour, we shared gentle laughter, a few highlights of Alabama football, and a prayer of gratefulness that he had survived the accident.

On the drive home that evening, I raged over the unfairness of what had happened. I could not imagine this vibrant young man in a wheelchair for the rest of his life. And yet I also felt a surprising calmness, an unexpected certainty that greater things were on the horizon for TJ and his family.

Two weeks later, I sat with TJ's Aunt Sandra watching an elementary school football game. She told me about his decision to participate in Geron's stem cell clinical trial, that it was a scientific landmark, and what it meant, not just for TJ, but for millions, if it turned out to be a success. For an hour we spoke as quietly as we could about TJ's bravery in agreeing to be the first human candidate in this study. We had both been reassured by Anita's latest update stating that he was doing extremely well considering everything he had been through. In the softest whisper, Sandra said that so far, there was no evidence that TJ's body was rejecting the cells or that he was experiencing any side effects. And then, before the horn sounded to end the fourth quarter, Sandra put her arm around my shoulder and whispered the seven words that shifted my life in a different direction: "I think you should write this story."

I looked into Sandra's face. Her eyes had a shining quickness that held me, commanding me to pause and reflect when my first reaction would have been to wrinkle my nose and shake my head "no" as in, *You've got to be kidding.* Instead, the swirling activity on the field and the spectators' cheers fell away, and my thoughts slid back into memory, as though Sandra's proposal had given them a starting push. She, somehow, believed my past experiences had put me in the right place at the right time to help TJ share this incredible story.

Sandra had known my extended family for longer than I. She had watched me grow up in rural Alabama with loving, hardworking parents who had strong beliefs in God and did their best to instill core values in our family. My dad was a respected politician and civic leader, a Mason of our community, and a deacon at Millry Baptist Church where my mother played the piano every Wednesday evening and for both Sunday services. Mother had a deep love for children and spent more than two decades as a teacher. English was by far her favorite subject. I believe she passed that on to me, and from my dad, I inherited his passion for documenting what was real, and tangible, in the world around us.

A small-town, church-centered childhood has a certain ineluctable grace. Although I had dreamed of being a pianist like my mother, I found great pleasure in playing the flute and participated in concert band during off seasons of volleyball and cheerleading. As the youngest of three children, I grew up idolizing my handsome, athletic big brother Brandon, and my sister Tera, the Goddess, who was four years older than me. She was everything I aspired to be: beautiful, kind, and loving. A stunning majorette, Tera was also in the top ten of her class academically. I felt so lucky to claim her, and this family, as mine.

But just before Christmas break 1987, Tera came to Mom and Dad and showed them an odd bump that had popped up on the front of her left ankle. Trying not to seem alarmed, Mom reached down and ran her fingers across Tera's ankle. A day later, she took Tera to our family physician, Dr. Paul Petcher, who told her to keep an eye on it. But when it failed to go away weeks later, Dr. Petcher wanted to perform a biopsy just to be sure the growth was nothing more than a ganglion cyst. Instead, the results pitched out our worst fear. At the age of fifteen, my sister Tera had a rare and deadly cancer called rhabdomyosarcoma.

What happened next was a progression of surgeries and chemotherapy, and a short-lived remission, as the cancer cells traveled aggressively from Tera's left leg and ankle to the lower lobe of her lung. Tera and Mom made the trip back to Birmingham for a new surgery and a more aggressive chemotherapy that wiped out her entire immune system and caused Tera to lose all of her beautiful dark hair. A feeling of absolute helplessness invaded me. I was just eleven and terribly frightened. Why was this happening to Tera, of all people? What had she ever done to deserve to be so sick and uncertain of her future? I asked these questions each day. No one had to tell me Tera was now fighting for her life. It all happened so quickly.

At her lowest, Tera weighed less than eighty pounds and her veins were ripped open beneath her skin. She was dying, and none of us could do anything but watch her suffer. Her blood counts were dropping precipitously, and my parents were advised to begin planning for her funeral. Our town initiated a prayer chain, which soon became a statewide effort, while our church family and schoolmates collected money so my parents could take off from work and travel to the hospital and be with Tera.

But Mom was relentless and would not resign herself to watching Tera die. She brought back one of my sister's earlier doctors, Dr. Dearth, who immediately wrote the order for Tera to be given total protein nutrient (TPN) treatments in conjunction with aggressive chemotherapy treatments. To date, that experimental cocktail had only been tested on a few patients, but the results were very promising. In less than two days, my parents saw improvement in Tera's energy level, and she was able to keep food and liquids down for more than twenty-four hours. The new protocol in fact worked like magic and helped Tera gain weight and strength to endure the chemotherapy treatments.

During his long career at Children's Hospital in Birmingham, Dr. Dearth had never seen a patient in Tera's condition recover so quickly after being given the TPN. He, too, a person of faith, believed wholeheartedly that prayers from our family, friends, and strangers across our state and beyond had made a difference in Tera's recovery and given her a second chance at life. But the science was indisputable. TPN, this new, still-being-tested elixir of a wonder drug, had been the key that saved my sister's life.

Now, as I sat along the turf of another grassy football field, I remembered how in May 1991, three and a half years after her diagnosis, Tera had walked across the field of our high school football stadium to proudly receive her diploma. My sister was a walking miracle and hero to many, myself included. Fast-forward twenty-three years to a house filled with mud-splattered baseball uniforms from her three sons, and a doting husband who adored her every move. Tera's life in the years since had been full and happy. But today her strength and inspiration became mine.

As I listened to Sandra talk about the stem cell treatment designed to, hopefully, regenerate damaged spinal cord tissue, I thought about Tera's TPN, the nutrients that back then were also experimental, that strengthened her so her body could accept the medication that would finally defeat her cancer. And I thought about the polycystic kidney disease I had, and that my children might inherit, where there were no known cures, yet. And my thoughts turned to TJ, a young man in the prime of his life who faced a future in a wheelchair, and who had said *Yes* to life, for himself, and possibly for millions.

Chance and faith. Medicine and miracles. Health and opportunity. These are among the balancing laws of nature. Didn't everyone deserve a shot at a full life?

My marriage of ten years over, my first novel treading water, I was ready for a new challenge. And I would be helping others in the process. I knew very little about the science behind embryonic stem cell research, but the church's position was immutable. Stem cells aroused great ire and opposition, but this was very different. I would have to teach myself, become a greater advocate, and negotiate controversy, all while making sure my family was protected.

I believe that everything has a season, and that we are guided by a higher law. The confluence of time, memory, and moment were right. I took Sandra's hand and smiled back at her. I would give this project my all.

With my heart and mind racing, I made a quick drive to my parents' home to seek counsel from the man I trusted most, my dad. For over an hour, I caught him up with TJ's transfer to the Shepherd Center, and his participation in the Geron trial. What Dad wanted to hear most, however, was why I felt compelled to help TJ with his story.

As most fathers are protective of their daughters' interests, Dad advised me to research the pros and cons of becoming involved with this controversial trial and, also, to make certain that my family and I would not be compromised or put in harm's way. Overall, Dad was supportive of the idea and encouraged me to move forward if my heart felt 100 percent committed to the project.

Following several phone conversations and email exchanges, Anita and TJ invited me to visit their family at the Shepherd Center in Atlanta. I arrived on Sunday, October 17, with another bag filled with snacks and get-well cards painted by my children.

TJ's identity as the research trial's first participant had not been revealed, and his medical team treated him no differently than any other patient. He seemed nervous, though, as if it had finally set in that he was the first person to receive these magic cells, the hope and focus of so many. Trying to ease his nerves, I sat on the edge of his bed and began sharing small funny stories about my children and their mischievous behavior over the past weekend. Sensing we were ready for private time to discuss the book project, Anita grabbed her purse and excused herself from the room.

Over the next three hours, TJ and I brainstormed the ways in which we might document his story of being the first patient in Geron's clinical trial. We tossed around the idea of publishing a shorter piece, perhaps a feature article in a major consumer scientific journal, but it seemed impossible to consolidate the scientific, religious, and political issues surrounding this trial. We agreed that with so many different angles and audiences to address, a chapter book was really the only way to portray the story. The longer we talked, the more excited TJ became about the new project. He was hopeful that when the timing was right for him to reveal his identity to the world, this story would change the hearts and minds of those who opposed stem cell treatment.

While TJ had dreamed of helping others through a nursing career, the uncertainty of achieving this goal, now from a wheelchair, stirred other options for a future for him in the medical industry. Through his story, he hoped to educate patients about the importance of clinical trials and how they can lead to the best treatments available—including the potential benefits of human embryonic stem cell therapy. TJ asked if I was willing to give everything I could to encourage the support for this crucial research. I assured him that I was behind him and progressive medicine 100 percent. I would carry this message of hope, healing, and determination with all of my heart.

There were tears in both our eyes. TJ's experience had already carried him beyond his young age. Lying in this bed had shaken up his sweetly ordered contentedness. From the purposeful look on his face and the calmness in his voice, I believed that he had chosen me to write this story for a reason. TJ knew that I was willing to go the extra mile and would never compromise the respect and dedication of those who had worked tirelessly to make this trial a reality. He knew that I would push forward regardless of the pressures or the resistance we encountered from others. We would be a good team.

TJ and I related to one another's pains and sufferings in life and understood when the other said, "Sometimes you just have to make the best of a bad situation and find a way to move forward!" We got that life moved relentlessly forward and was most satisfyingly spent helping as many people as possible along the way. Above all, we thanked God for giving us strength to persevere.

Before making the trip back home to Millry, I left TJ a note of encouragement with words written from Ralph Waldo Emerson: "For everything you have missed, you have gained something else; and for everything you gain, you lose something else. . . . You can either regret or rejoice. The choice is yours."

A few weeks later, a wonderful opportunity appeared that would help both my family and also TJ's story. On November 16, I was hired by a rural electric utility company as editor of their in-house magazine and as the cooperative's communication specialist. This new position gave me great experience in public speaking, working with tight deadlines, connecting with others in the publishing industry, and learning how to maximize social media. It also allowed me to build a network of professionals who were willing and able to assist in any capacity—all tools the months and years ahead would require of me in abundance.

I embraced this opportunity and felt certain God had opened another door to help bring this story to life.

9

AN INSIDE LOOK

Menlo Park, California
October 2010–October 2011

As the Geron team prepared to leave Atlanta, it was a relief for them to know that everything had gone well with their first injection of GRNOPC1. However, Geron's medical director, Dr. Ed Wirth, worried whether it was possible for nine more patients to meet all of the inclusion criteria for the study. En route to the West Coast, he and his team felt an intense urgency to get all the other clinical sites ready to enroll patients. The entire team was committed and agreed to be on call 24/7 until nine additional patients were enrolled in Phase 1.

With less than 2 percent of all newly injured spinal cord injury patients anticipated to meet the eligibility criteria of age, level of injury, and healthy immune systems—and among these, much fewer choosing to participate—Ed knew it would be extremely tough enrolling eight patients, but not impossible.

From his recruitment to Geron in 2004 until the trial began in 2010, Ed had spent an enormous amount of time researching potential trial locations and building strong relationships with top hospital administrators. He spoke with approximately forty spinal cord injury hospitals and rehabilitation centers across the United States about participating in the trial and was determined to have the selected sites functional before the end of 2011. With Atlanta's Shepherd Center and Northwestern University in Chicago already active sites, these remaining seven centers would soon be functional sites as well: University of Alabama at Birmingham located in Birmingham, Alabama; Stanford University located in Palo Alto, California; Santa Clara Valley Medical Center in San Jose, California; University of Maryland Medical Center and Kernan Orthopaedics & Rehabilitation Hospital located in Baltimore, Maryland; Thomas Jefferson University Hospital located in Philadelphia, Pennsylvania; and The Medical College of Wisconsin located in Milwaukee, Wisconsin.

But selecting these study locations was not a simple task for Ed and his team. Using the U.S. Census as a resource to guide him to the key trauma centers, Ed pushed on. He quickly realized there was a major setback with this approach: as the census revealed, most spinal cord injuries did not occur in the larger metro areas. The majority of these injuries originated in rural areas and were often associated with high speed car accidents, motorcycle accidents, significant falls from climbing accidents, and swimming accidents. This made enrollment for the trial extremely challenging for Geron because local hospitals were treating most of these accident victims, not trauma centers.

For these reasons, Ed consulted with Linda Jones, Geron's clinical trial coordinator, and they considered hiring a recruiting company to help locate eligible patients. Early into their search, they learned that most companies did not network with smaller, rural hospitals, which would therefore decrease the odds of patients being transported to larger hospitals in time to be screened for the trial.

From a feasibility perspective, the protocol specified that patients had to live no more than 120 miles away from one of the study centers. Ed felt this was extremely limiting, so he encouraged Geron to work with each study center on a case-by-case basis when considering accepting patients from any location in the lower forty-eight states. When the trial was ready to start in July 2010, Geron's CEO Tom Okarma and senior management had agreed with Ed, and decided that Geron would pay for the patient's ground or air ambulance transport, if needed, to get to the study center for evaluation. Also in the agreement, Geron would pay for the patient's return trip home if he or she did not qualify.

Considering these issues, Ed was not surprised that it took several months to get the trial up and running. In August, just days after Northwestern University opened as the first study center, Ed received a call that a patient had been screened and met all inclusion criteria.

Andy Bridge was injured on August 22, 2010, when he fell three flights and fractured his spine at T5–6. After surgery, Andy was diagnosed as a complete T4 spinal cord injury with no health issues other than his acute injury. About five days postop, Andy's surgeon, Dr. Liu, offered him the choice to be the first patient to receive Geron's stem cell transplant.

Andy, also a physician, was able to make an informed decision based on his own medical knowledge. Putting science aside, he felt a decision of this magnitude was monumental, life-changing not only for himself but possibly for millions around the globe. He did not believe there was a right or wrong decision, but only a decision that was right in his heart. Just hours leading up to surgery, Andy withdrew his name from the list and chose not to be injected with stem cells.

Indeed, there was a long wait between Andy Bridge and TJ Atchison, which included another upset just a few weeks later at Shepherd Center in Atlanta when the unidentified Patient X withdrew from the trial just hours before surgery in fear of the science involved in the protocol. To make matters worse, Ed expected it to be even more difficult to enroll patients from November until February, because fewer spinal cord injuries occur during the winter months. So Ed took advantage of the fallow time to work on a grant application for $25 million from the California Institute of Regenerative Medicine (CIRM) to help fund the next several phases of the trial, including the start-up and several tweaks of the protocol itself.

CIRM had been established six years before, in 2004, when California voters used Dr. Hans Keirstead's groundbreaking research as an example of the promise of human embryonic stem cell therapies in the run-up to a vote for Proposition 71. This $3 billion bond initiative passed by a wide margin and amended the state constitution by creating a new source of research funding in California. The dream of a public-private cooperation became a working reality and closed the critical funding gap created by Bush-era federal policy that prevented the rapid advancement of stem cell research that could help millions in California. CIRM in fact became a force and a model for public-private partnerships that kept researchers in California, while driving the economy, creating jobs, building infrastructure, and attracting young, talented researchers to the West Coast.

Most importantly, Ed believed the funds from this grant would allow Geron to expand the number of cells in the initial injection dosage to a higher level that his team felt would be more optimal for showing functional recovery, around twenty million cells. Before the trial was originally approved in July, the FDA demanded that Geron start with just two million stem cells, a figure Ed and his team believed straddled the lower ends of the efficacy range. However, to keep the trial moving forward, Geron agreed to this low dosage and felt it was acceptable for both ethical and safety reasons. If the trial were to successfully move beyond Phase 1, Ed would increase the dosage to five to ten times higher in Phases 2, 3, and 4.

The CIRM grant came down to the wire for Geron, as no one from the biotech company had been in touch with CIRM representatives nor had the company heard any updates from the grant review board. This silence alarmed Ed, so he put in a call to a friend, the patient advocate Roman Reed. After Roman became paralyzed in a college football accident in 1994, he became the driver and inspiration behind a California bill that passed in 1999, the Roman Reed Spinal Cord Injury Research Act. In fact, Dr. Hans Keirstead's original research at UC-Irvine was funded through "Roman's Law," which led to the paralysis breakthrough discovery that Geron bought in 2001.

Ed asked Roman if he and his father Don Reed, who served on the executive board for Proposition 71 and supported grassroots efforts across the state for stem cell research, would write CIRM's grant review board a letter of support for the Geron trials. Roman and Don, both very much respected in the stem cell community and true champions for the field of regenerative medicine, were eager to help.

Roman and Don immediately each wrote compelling letters on Geron's behalf, and also attended CIRM's public meeting to personally voice their support for funding its clinical trial. Nonetheless, the vote was close. Advocates representing other neurological diseases like Parkinson's and Alzheimer's had asked for funding too, and there were skeptics on the grant committee who felt that Geron was moving too far, too soon into unchartered territory with their clinical trial.

Don waited patiently for his one minute at the microphone and shared, through his and Roman's unique perspectives, why a trial like this should be funded. He said, "On March 1, 2002, at the Reeve-Irvine Research Center, Roman and I witnessed Dr. Keirstead's amazing research. We held in our hands a formerly paralyzed rat called Fighter and believed that maybe, just maybe, because of what happened that day, there would become a time when Roman, too, would walk again." Don looked at each member of the panel and said, "Please fund this trial so that paralysis is no longer a life sentence for my son or for millions of others."

Bob Klein, founder and chairman of CIRM, who had a son with type 1 diabetes, also advocated for Geron and provided credibility that all appropriate steps had been taken by the biotech company to resolve all safety and ethical issues. He expressed the importance of Dr. Keirstead's embryonic stem cell therapy moving toward human clinical trials.

The summer and fall of 2011 was an important period for Ed and his team. Geron was awarded the $25 million grant they sought from CIRM, which meant that $45 million had now been invested into the stem cell clinical trial. In addition, a second and then a third patient were enrolled in the study, followed by the first two patients from the West Coast, making a total of five patients enrolled in the trial. Little by little, Geron was putting together the pieces that would get the trial going full steam. Ed Wirth and Linda Jones were thrilled to be enrolling patients at a quicker pace and optimistic of meeting their goal of eight to ten patients before year's end.

Now, as he anticipated Phase 2 beginning in January 2012, Ed was very eager to escalate the cell dosage up to the range he felt would be optimal for therapeutic results. But behind closed doors, there was much discord between Geron's senior management and its board of directors. Regardless of the positive outcome measures being reported from the safety study data from Geron, the board had different plans for their expensive stem cell program, involving in fact, shutting it down completely. This action spelled the end of CEO Tom Okarma's golden reign, as he was forced out of the biotech company. Then, Geron announced it was through with regenerative medicine altogether, putting an end to active research programs on three major cell types for therapies—neural, cardiac, and pancreatic.

Ed understood the company's restructuring from a business perspective, but he couldn't understand why Geron would choose to shake things up when there were three major studies under way, including an oncology operation that was a Phase 1 study of a licensed compound, and most recently, GRNOPC1. Ed and his team sensed that the stem cell program just getting started was going to prove to be too expensive for too long. Their hunch was confirmed a month after Okarma's departure, when the newly appointed CEO, David Greenwood, justified the board's decision by stating that, without these changes, the company would be spending at least $25 million per year on its stem cell efforts over the next few years.

A company the size of Geron, already in competition with a competing cancer program, would not be able to underwrite two big programs. The economy had tumbled with the 2008 recession, and without having solid results to show, the company's stock price was flat. So after the CIRM funding was awarded, Geron announced it would commit $8 million to wind down the spinal cord injury study and follow the five transplanted patients with periodic assessments for fifteen years.

This news was both disturbing and disappointing for Northwestern's lead investigator, Dr. Richard Fessler, as he and the other investigators had placed an inordinate amount of time, resources, and trust in Geron.

It was dishearteningly obvious to Ed and his colleagues that Geron was restructuring to be solely an oncology clinical trial company. Indeed, the new management group was already beginning to dismantle the senior team that had guided GRNOPC1 to its current stage.

Expecting the stem cell research trials at Geron to come to an end, Ed explained to the few remaining team members that there were two types of research: cutting-edge and bleeding-edge. Cutting-edge research consisted of novel breakthroughs that could be predicted and strategically planned. Unfortunately, the GRNOPC1 protocol fell into the bleeding-edge research category, in that this unpredictable study would face many setbacks along the way, including not having enough money to complete the trial.

And so by September 2011, Ed realized he didn't have a team any longer and that it was time for him to move on too. As it became increasingly clear that the stem cell program at Geron was over, Ed also feared other companies would henceforth be more reluctant to follow their footsteps. There were dozens of companies, mostly start-ups, working on potential stem cell treatments; the news at Geron could cause another major setback for the entire field of regenerative medicine.

Accepting what he could not change, Ed took out his Rolodex and began making calls. He was fortunate that Frank Reynolds, CEO of In-Vivo Therapeutics, a company focused on the development of groundbreaking technologies for the treatment of spinal cord injuries, badly wanted him to serve as their new chief scientific officer. So in early October, Ed turned in his notice but stayed on with Geron to celebrate the one-year anniversary of the stem cell clinical trial launch, and also because he very much wanted to see the image results from study day 365.

Based on animal studies, the Geron team knew that injected cells of GRNOPC1 could potentially migrate or move into normal spinal cord tissue beyond the injury zone. The concerns of this migration causing any harm or unexpected neurological symptoms had been resolved in additional animal studies, but Ed and his researchers were still responsible for monitoring all patients for this and other possible risks of GRNOPC1.

Ed's greatest concern was the risk of patients developing cells that produced fluid, which could put pressure on the spinal cord and cause further damage. The chances were small that any fluid-filled cystic structures would develop, but were this to occur, Ed was certain the FDA would no longer support embryonic stem cell research and deem the technology unsafe for human therapy.

Although Ed was not a board-certified radiologist, he had reviewed enough MRI readings in his twenty years to know what to look for and make certain the radiologist was reading them accurately.

To further monitor the study images, Ed and his study team at Geron hired a company that specialized in working with clinical trial sites to electronically upload the MRI images from the study centers to the company's servers. The imaging company provided several services for Geron, including guaranteeing the images were obtained according to protocol and that they self-maintained a call schedule with a radiologist who was trained on the protocol and who could read, discuss, and sign off on the electronic documentation of results. Thus, after every MRI was obtained from the study, Ed received notification by Web interface and could log into the image-reading software and review the images privately.

Right through Ed's final days at Geron, there had been no evidence that any fluid-filled cystic structures had occurred or additional damage to the spinal cord noted. It would take about five years postinjection for patients to be considered out of the woods, but at 365 days postop injection, Ed felt confident his five patients would experience no adverse affects from GRNOPC1. In this, the clinical trial would be deemed a success.

With a new position waiting for him at InVivo Therapeutics, Ed could look forward to new research challenges ahead. He would never quite understand why Geron did not stay on track with the stem cell study. It was a profound disappointment to him, given the enormous amount of time and the financial investment that had been pumped into the GRNOPC1. But there was nothing more he could do to convince senior management differently. He was determined to advance the study of stem cell research, and felt his future at another company would contribute to other breakthroughs that would make a huge impact. For TJ, Roman Reed, and the other men and women living with disease and injury, that crack of hope would have to suffice for now.

10

THE HUMAN CANDIDATE

Jackson, Alabama, and Atlanta, Georgia
October 2010–March 2011

Switching gears from writing my young adult story to writing solely about the Geron trials, I felt a bit uneasy about abandoning my first book but made a vow to return to it after making this new project a success. With research consuming every spare second of each day, I began to draft a book proposal after the children's bedtime and during my lunch break at work. The small, quaint, rural town of Jackson, Alabama, where my job was located was the perfect place to pull out of my daily routine and focus on this new story. My favorite spot to write was a bluff overlooking the Tombigbee River where I parked my car under the tender protection of a large shade tree. Here, I happily escaped into my writing.

My social life necessarily dwindled down to work-related activities and family lunch on Sunday. There was no time for anything but work, children, and writing. My friends were growing frustrated, too, and often complained about my busy schedule. The few that truly knew my heart understood that my top priorities were taking care of my children and meeting writing deadlines. Only a handful of intimates knew that I was working quietly to create a book proposal for this story. But living as I did in such a small town, several others were becoming suspicious and asked why I was making so many weekend trips to Atlanta. My response was always the same, "Just keeping Anita company while TJ's in rehab at the Shepherd Center."

On Friday, November 12, the children and I drove a few miles to TJ's family home in Chatom and picked up his younger brother Tucker. We had planned a road trip to visit TJ and Anita, and asked Tucker to make the trip with us to surprise his family. It was an emotional trip for Tucker and me, as we spent most of the seven-hour drive talking about his love for TJ and how he prayed each day that his big brother would walk again. I shared with Tucker the story of my sister's battle with cancer. I understood how much it hurt to watch someone you love suffer and not be able to do anything about it. I encouraged Tucker to continue praying and supporting his family, and assured him that they were a strong group who could make it through this difficult time.

We arrived at the Shepherd Center at 3 p.m. and witnessed a tearful reunion between TJ, Anita, and Tucker. My children smothered Anita with hugs and kisses, and then pounced all over her daughter Alyssa, who is the same age as my twins, Carlie and Conner. Our families had spent countless playdates and birthday celebrations together over the course of five years. We were as close as friends could be, and depended on each other during life's ups and downs.

That evening, we took Anita and Alyssa for a little break away from the rehab center and let Tucker and TJ have some private time. We drove thirty miles north to Alpharetta to Georgia's American Girl store, arriving there just before dusk. We pulled into the parking lot and saw a beautiful carousel spinning inside the atrium. For the next few hours, we did our best to alleviate Anita's and Alyssa's sadness with a fun-filled evening of shopping, fantasy, and laughter.

December 2010 came and went, with my children's father making an appearance the week of Christmas to say his final good-byes and pack up the remainder of his personal belongings. He had decided to move nearly two hours away from us to Sumter County, offering no explanation, which made it extremely difficult for the children and me to find peace and closure. With the new year just ahead, I resolved to move forward with confidence in raising my children as a single parent.

By January 4, 2011, I had completed a first draft of the proposal for the book we were then calling "The Human Candidate" and began querying literary agents with a one-page pitch letter:

Dear Mr./Ms. Agent:

On September 25, 2010, a close friend of my family was injured in a terrible automobile accident that left him paralyzed from the chest down. One week following his accident, he was transferred to the Shepherd Center in Atlanta, Georgia, and became the first spinal cord injury patient to be injected with human embryonic stem cells. My project, The Human Candidate, is a story that captures the beauty and drama of scientific discovery, as well as the selfless determination of many to help millions of disabled people across the globe.

Hope is found in this inspiring true story of the recipient, the victim of an automobile accident that left him paralyzed from the chest down when he was only twenty-one years old. As the first patient with a spinal cord injury to be injected with human embryonic stem cells, he courageously tells the story of his life and healing, in a work that will resonate far beyond being the human candidate that made medical history.

Sorely interested in this remarkable clinical trial, I agreed to help the recipient convert his story into a documentary that would enlighten other young people as well as adults as to exactly what is involved with the use of embryonic stem cell therapy. Not only has the recipient provided dozens of photos to include in this story, but he has also given photocopies of privileged information and allowed me to record interviews that have taken place since his accident in September. A contract declaring me as author-in-full has been signed and is available per your request.

I am the editor for Clarke-Washington EMC's magazine, *Alabama Living*, with a circulation of 22,000 customers in southwest Alabama each month. I hope you are interested in seeing my proposal, and if so, I would be most happy to send this material to you as soon as possible . . .

Because this story was a nonfiction project based on real people and events, I could not submit the proposal to the same literary agents to whom I had queried my young adult book. Each agent specialized according to his or her own literary interest and typically did not cross genres unless his or her client already had an established readership or was a high-profile celebrity.

The query process was extremely challenging for "The Human Candidate" because I did not feel comfortable revealing TJ's identity, nor sharing specifics about the clinical trial to anyone. I respected the privacy issues for all involved and understood the importance of keeping information about the trial privileged and away from the public eye until TJ felt comfortable revealing his identity.

So with my query letters out, I waited anxiously for a response. In the meantime, I began the next phase of my book research, the validation from witnesses, researchers, and experts in the biotech community willing to flesh out the details in this story. That began a cross-country search to reach out to the experts who had contributed to developing GRNOPC1, and to the patient advocates who had raised awareness and funding for this novel research approach.

I started in February 2011 with the medical director for the Shepherd Center, Dr. Donald Leslie, who graciously agreed to meet with me. It wasn't long after arriving at the rehab center that I realized how busy Monday mornings were for everyone—patients filled the waiting areas and staff members moved purposefully about. With very few vacant chairs in the lobby area and an hour to spare before my appointment with Dr. Leslie, I began wandering up and down the hallways of the Shepherd Center. This was now my sixth visit to the center, and I was amazed that I had somehow overlooked a wall filled with beautiful artwork. Most of the pieces were painted by former patients. There were also awards recognizing the achievements of staff and administrators, and there were photographs commemorating the center's thirty-five-year history.

Minutes later, a security officer passed and asked if I needed help finding my way. I suppose the large duffel bag of notebooks and reference books I carried was a sure giveaway I was not there for medical reasons. I explained that I was waiting to interview Dr. Leslie, and mentioned that I would love to find a quiet place to write. She smiled and pointed me in the direction of the Noble Learning Resource Center, which was just down the hallway and to the left.

In the few steps it took to reach the library, I passed a couple standing near a young man, their son it appeared, in a wheelchair, and inadvertently overheard their conversation. Suddenly the memories of TJ's experience as a patient at the facility just months before quickly came back to me. I heard the same determination and strength in this family's conversation as I had heard then, and I realized these same events and moments—as uncertainty met reality, and of being young and disabled—replayed themselves with fresh force.

It was in fact this unexpected encounter, combined with my two-hour interview with Dr. Leslie, that led to a rush of ideas that filled over a dozen pages that evening. As I wrote from my hotel room on Peachtree Street, the intensity of the words I penned was unlike that of any others

I had produced. Dr. Leslie's interview was still fresh on my mind, particularly these words of truth: "It is about outcomes; it is about people's lives and how people's lives change in an instant with their injury," that subtly shifted the axis of my intent. With Dr. Leslie's final words, "You're the perfect person to share this story," I realized that I was no longer writing for TJ alone, but for millions of other patients who pray each day for a cure for disease or injury. At the heart of it all, it was the family at Shepherd and Dr. Leslie who helped me realize that my mission for "The Human Candidate" was to educate an entire planet on the benefits of regenerative medicine and to encourage all to support stem cell research.

11

BRIDGING THE GAP BETWEEN SCIENCE AND RELIGION

Millry, Alabama
March–June 2011

Two weeks later, on March 25, 2011, a wonderful literary agent, Mac Mackie of Old North Literary in North Carolina, responded to my proposal and requested a phone call the following day to discuss a potential offer of agent representation. I was elated that Mac—someone with no direct relationship with spinal cord injury or with a medical background—connected with both the human interest aspect of the story and its importance to evolving science. This was validation of a different sort, that my proposal for "The Human Candidate" could in fact become a published book and educate many on the importance of stem cell research.

For nearly an hour, I sat inside my car in the office parking lot and listened to Mac's every word as if my life hinged on the conversation. I knew I would learn a lot from Mac and that he would guide me through the process of developing this proposal into a completed book. He felt confident that we could editorially polish the content, place it with the right editor, and make the best book possible. Those were the pragmatics, but Mac also felt that he could help me achieve the goal of furthering awareness and promotion of stem cell research across the Bible Belt region as part of a larger effort to inform and help future generations to come.

And so two days later, on March 28, 2011, Mac officially made an offer to represent both me and TJ on "The Human Candidate." TJ and I talked by phone that evening and emailed Mac the following day, accepting his offer of agent representation.

One week later, TJ and I announced the book project on my blog, and received a flood of interest and support from people across the globe. Robert "Bob" Stein, the chief science editor at the *Washington Post* called and explained he was writing a story about the progress of the Geron trials, then still very much under way. He asked if I would share information about TJ and his decision to participate in the study. I admired Bob's writing and journalistic approach in covering hot-topic issues, and felt flattered he was interested in my perspective. I was definitely interested and willing to help, but at that very moment, with the kids splashing soapy water in my eyes as we tried to bathe our puppy, I asked if he would call again the next day.

It was becoming more and more difficult balancing family life with the increased activity and interest stemming from this new venture. My stress was building as well, but the more interest the project received, the better I became at dealing with it. I discovered there were no more satisfying phrases for a writer than "Please speak to my agent" and "No comment." In many situations, these were truly words of beauty.

Just before bed, I had researched Bob enough to know that he was brilliant at tearing down fences that protected off-limit topics to the general public. He was also very clever at making everything available, which terrified me that I would say too much about TJ and the clinical trial. I emailed Mac and TJ and requested a morning call to discuss Bob's request to interview me for his article.

During our teleconference, we agreed to allow the *Post* an exclusive interview, but felt it was in the best interest of the book that all other interviews (newspapers and television) take place after "The Human Candidate" was scheduled to debut. Our writing team was appreciative of the positive interest and felt confident Bob's piece would be important to help get our message out. God willing, our proposal would evolve into a completed book very soon.

When the appointed hour arrived, Bob immediately picked up on my wide-eyed innocence and probed gently for as much information as he could get regarding TJ's progress since the stem cell injection. Again, not trying to sound rude, I explained as politely as I could that I was not at liberty to disclose specifics about the trial or TJ's progress, although

I was happy to share general information about our book project. As I shared my passion for documenting this story, Bob said, "You know, I think what you and TJ are trying to accomplish through this book is great. And it sounds like you are persistent enough to make it happen."

Bob's encouragement was very uplifting and propelled me to press forward. He was most interested in my religious perspective, and asked if my position on the issue of stem cell research had changed since beginning this new adventure with TJ.

At this point in the interview, there was no tension or nervousness, which allowed me to relax and feel comfortable in my response. I explained that when I decided to write TJ's story, I anticipated there would be ethical implications requiring serious consideration. My parents were also concerned that I was stepping into controversial territory and that the blowback—from friends, from our Baptist church, and from our conservative community—could be hurtful. As I became privy to information and constrained by confidentiality agreements, I knew that I would be thrust into the limelight and targeted by those who opposed stem cell research.

When TJ and I decided to go public with this project, as people heard and learned about it from my blog and other social media sources, I saw it was indeed a minefield and a place where there was as much honestly held conviction as there was confusion, and that science, scripture, tradition, and geography certainly clashed. I kept asking myself *Why derail other writing projects to subject my family and me to uncomfortable situations and accusations?* But my answer was simple: to make a real difference in this world.

There were more positive comments than negative being made about the project in public and across the Internet, but it was difficult not responding to messages like these: "Tory and TJ are promoting abortion through this story," and "I'd hate to see what happens to her [Me] for revealing classified information in this excitement."

As these comments went straight into our trash folders, I focused on the difference our efforts were making in the lives of so many, and that reward and motivation made me embrace the project even more. I had the privilege of helping shift public opinion on stem cell research, and of making a difference for regenerative medicine. This knowledge kept me going during many frustrating times. I came to understand there was room for daylight too—where people could agree to disagree and move beyond the stem cell debate with respect of one another's positions. And

I found a personal place of peace and understanding that allowed me to commit myself with a clear conscience.

The following day, I learned through a friend that Bob had also interviewed TJ's preacher, Brother Troy Bailey. It would not be until the piece ran on April 15, 2011, that Bailey would learn that his words had led to controversy. From Bob's thirty-five-minute interview with Bailey, probably less than 2 percent of what the Pentecostal preacher had said was included in the final article, titled "Stem Cells Were God's Will, Says First Recipient of Treatment."

Because of these few, brief quotes of Bailey's, edited and printed out of context, he was later called everything from a simpleton to a Nazi: "I am adamantly against abortion in any form. It did cause me some searching and researching biblically of what is the proper answer. I don't really see a baby's life was destroyed for this to take place. I'm definitely not wanting to encourage harvesting embryos for all kinds of crazy reasons, and that definitely led some people to have some hesitancy about some of these things."

Brother Bailey felt strong in his convictions and had no issue sharing what he believed. He was convinced that Bob Stein was really seeking to juice up the controversial aspects of the issue. Bailey later said that he was disappointed that this important quote never made it to print in Bob's article: "Personally, I feel that it's being on God's side of the issue that matters most."

On June 15, 2011, I also had the opportunity to interview Brother Bailey. Meeting inside his pastoral study at Reynolds Holiness Church, he clearly explained that he saw the issue as both more certain and more complex than partisans on either side of the debate allowed. To begin, he did not support human cloning or embryonic stem cell research, and he worried the potential risks—like people losing sight of the sacredness of these cells—could outweigh the benefits. But on one point he was clear: he had never, ever advised anyone on the subject of embryonic stem cells, including TJ, who had already made his decision to participate in the stem cell trial and had given his written consent to proceed before Bailey was ever even informed.

He explained to me, "Even a cursory look at scripture shows that God condemns murder; a closer look at scripture reveals that life begins at conception, not at birth. With this in mind, it is evident to me that abortion is murder."

To engage me in the discussion, he asked, "What is your definition of conception? What does it mean to conceive?"

Before I could voice my thoughts, Bailey answered, "For every doctor or medical text that can be cited as defining conception as the moment of fertilization, another can be quoted as defining it as the moment of implantation. Biblically, to conceive is to be pregnant or 'with child.' Therefore, only women are said to conceive."

In this framework, he believed that when an ovum became released by a woman's body it was an independent cell and was no longer a part of her body. To validate his theory, he explained, "When the ovum is fertilized it is still independent of a woman's body, which is why fertilization can take place outside of her body. A woman conceives or becomes pregnant when one or more fertilized ovum implants in her uterus. It's at this point that the pregnancy test will register positive. God told Eve that He would multiply her sorrow and conception, referring to the pain and suffering of childbirth, but the pain and suffering are due to her pregnancy, not to the fertilization of an ovum that may never even result in a pregnancy."

I agreed with much of Brother Bailey's response: Life begins at conception in a woman's womb. But then, I wondered, when did a person's life begin? I asked him, "At what specific point does a person become a living soul?"

And he was quick to answer, "The Bible declares we are the creation of God and that He forms us in our mother's womb. Man may take the initial ingredients for life, mix them together in a petri dish, and proudly assert that he has created a human being; but in nine months you won't be able to cradle his creation, rock it to sleep, or say that it looks just like it's daddy because it'll still be nothing more than a blastocyst in a petri dish. Being a living soul is more than just possessing DNA."

Brother Bailey paused for a short moment, took out pen and paper, and then drew several diagrams which illustrated these points: "If one believes a fertilized ovum can split before implantation, then to say a person becomes a living soul at fertilization implies that a soul can split and become two souls, or two people can possess the same soul. Since we know that two fertilized ovums [before implantation] can combine and become one, while containing two DNA, then one must also conclude that two souls must be able to become one soul. As a matter of fact, one fertilized ovum can be split four ways in a lab, then be implanted in the uterus of one or more women and four identical twins can be born all with the same DNA."

With a soft smile across his face, Brother Bailey flipped the question around to me and asked, "So, does life begin at fertilization or does life begin at conception?"

I was about to respond, but again, he interjected before I could answer, "The Bible has much to say about the specific length or duration of our lives and even teaches us to number our days. Life must have a definite beginning and ending; a point when the clock starts ticking and a point when it stops. To say that a life can begin when two cells are fused together in a petri dish at a fertility clinic and are then preserved indefinitely in that state implies that life can begin and not end. However, once a fertilized ovum implants in a woman's womb, thereby starting a pregnancy, the clock starts, along with growth and development that can only be stopped by death."

Now this was a statement that resonated with me deeply. I wiped the sweat bubbles from my forehead and explained to Brother Bailey that six weeks into my second pregnancy, I began to experience intense pain. It was suspected that I could be miscarrying. My doctor arranged for me to return to the hospital early the next morning for a scan, but that night, the pain became severe. Calling my doctor, I was told I was in real trouble and to get to the hospital right away. I was having an ectopic pregnancy.

It took all my strength just to stagger to the car, and the forty-five-minute journey to Druid City Hospital in Tuscaloosa was a blur.

Once admitted, I was given morphine to ease the pain. The doctors tried to perform a scan, but my right fallopian tube was very swollen and minutes away from rupturing, which could cause severe life-threatening internal bleeding. My condition was critical and they decided to operate immediately. The last thing I remember was asking the doctor to please not remove any reproductive organs unless it was absolutely necessary for my survival.

When I came to from the operation, the agonizing pain had gone but I had to deal with the heartbreaking reality that it was a double loss—the pregnancy had failed and I had lost my right fallopian tube.

The doctors said I was lucky to be alive, but I felt crushed. There was nothing I could have done to prevent the ectopic pregnancy. There were many tear-filled days that followed. It honestly felt like the end of the world.

Everything happened so quickly I never had time to think about it until after my operation. Once I was discharged from the hospital I was left feeling very alone, with so many "what-ifs" running through my head. It was heartbreaking telling Catie that she would not have a baby brother or sister to play with.

Still wanting a second child, I was worried that I wouldn't be able to become pregnant again and felt frightened that if I did become pregnant, I might have another ectopic pregnancy. There were days when I wondered whether we should even try again, considering the risks of experiencing another ectopic pregnancy (7–10 percent). I didn't know if I could handle another failed pregnancy.

When I did become pregnant again, I was understandably anxious. At week six, an early scan reassured me, showing the baby safely attached in my womb. The first trimester came and went with zero morning sickness and with the telltale hormone levels perfect. After I had made it to the second trimester and passed the crucial tests, I decided to try to let go of the fear and embrace this pregnancy. Everything was going according to plan, and I was thrilled that our eighteenth-week ultrasound revealed we were having another baby girl. We were also excited to see real baby features aside from the blobs we had seen at earlier ultrasounds. We left the office glowing from excitement.

Then, a month later, at twenty-two weeks into the pregnancy, I felt something different. I knew the baby was growing more and more each day; in fact, I thought I had felt a little twinge of a foot or an arm pressing on my bladder. This feeling intensified into something very different from a moving and growing baby. I felt as if she had drifted more to my back, as if her weight was causing more pressure on my kidneys and intestines. There was no relief, and the pain was worsening. Finally, I knew something wasn't right and I asked my husband to take me to the emergency room.

The seventy-mile drive to Mobile was a nightmare. I could feel my body push and my husband kept asking me not to push if I could help it. I tried to stop my uterus from contracting but there was no control over the pushing. My daughter Sarah Margaret ("Maggie") was born seventeen weeks premature, and lived for just five days.

I looked over at Pastor Bailey and wiped a tear from my cheek. I explained that I did not expect to see a baby in Heaven from my ectopic pregnancy because this was simply a cluster of cells that had lodged in my fallopian tube. This cell cluster had never developed into a baby, therefore, I did not consider it to be a living soul.

As for my preterm baby Maggie, she was a living, breathing baby that had a head full of black hair, a beating heart, and had thrived inside my womb for more than twenty-two weeks. I had felt her move and hiccup and tumble inside my body for weeks before her preterm delivery. Maggie was a living soul and, yes, I would see her in Heaven.

So for me it was as clear as the skein of daylight. Life began not at fertilization, but rather at conception.

With tears also building in Brother Bailey's eyes, I asked his viewpoints on the use of oral contraceptives and on couples seeking help from reproductive centers. His response: "If one views the beginning of life to be at fertilization, then one must also be opposed to oral contraceptives since they can prevent the implanting of a fertilized ovum and thereby cause the destruction of a life." He continued, "One must also view fertility clinics with the same disdain as abortion clinics since unused, fertilized ova are being aborted by being thrown away in garbage bins. Even in the cases of those that aren't discarded, one must decide if it's morally right to create lives in a fertility clinic that won't all be given a chance to develop to birth and live their lives."

Brother Bailey expressed his greatest concern by posing this question, "How can we justify creating more embryos when there are an estimated 500,000 already being preserved in fertility clinics in the United States alone? Is there any difference in a woman purposely giving birth to triplets, picking out the one she wants to raise, and then leaving the others at the hospital not knowing if they're going to die or one day be adopted? I believe this answer to be 'No.' However, we, as a nation, will never prohibit couples from seeking reproductive assistance to have a family. Reproductive centers have helped so many couples to become parents and this is when I believe abandoned embryos, those doomed for garbage dumpsters, should be used to help people who are sick and dying."

I, too, had argued this exact point to close friends and family members during the early days following my announcement of helping TJ with this story. Many knew that I had gone through two years of fertility treatments to have my twins, and that I would have been crushed if I was denied this right to have more children after my ectopic pregnancy and losing my daughter Maggie. This was invariably the lightbulb moment, when my close friends and family realized that hESC research did not in fact destroy life, but that these sacred cells could be used to help millions who suffered from disease and injury and thus enhance life.

Brother Bailey further explained that it was not his personal style to write articles and condemnatory responses to controversial issues or to pass blanket judgments on people he'd never met. But he spoke of his respect and support for those who valiantly fight for the lives of the unborn and against the evils of abortion. He claimed that he fought for the same cause, but in his own way. As an older preacher once said to him, "Be careful, there's a ditch on both sides of the road!" Brother Bailey interpreted that message as meaning a driver can swerve to stay out of the ditch on the left side of the road and end up in the ditch on the right side of the road. Moral to the story: The driver should focus on the middle lines of the road, where it's safe.

I nodded my head as he made the point that it's one thing to fight for what's right, but sometimes we can carry the fight too far. "A doctor may have to apply the knife to remove a tumor," he continued, "and when he does we want him to get it all, but we sure don't want him to remove any more than is absolutely necessary. As a pastor, I have to deal up close and personal with people whose lives are being devastated by divorce, death, drug addiction, terminal illness, suicide, and paralysis, to name just a few."

Bailey believes in the authority of a moral compass that delineates what is right and wrong, no matter who it affects. But he also believes that when you're dealing every day with real people with very real hurts and pains, you tend to be a little more hesitant to pass quick judgment. Indeed, in his work, his instinct is to show support, as well as compassion, but he knows that life, and lives, are messy. So he's had to take stands and sometimes tell people things he knew they didn't want to hear. There were many times when he didn't get to say, "No comment" or get to pick and choose what he wanted to respond to. And then there are times when life seizes and spasms, and we are overwhelmed by its mysteries.

And so there have been times such as when Bailey had to hold the bloody hand of a teenager—in an emergency room, who's just been told he's lost his entire family—and know that his answers to the young man's questions could affect the rest of his life, or that a couple's young daughter will not survive long enough to enroll in an upcoming clinical trial that could cure her rare cancer.

So the bottom line for Brother Bailey was this: he wanted to have the courage to go as far as he had to in order to defend his truth, yet have the compassion not to go one step further than the truth demanded. "We must find a way to bridge the gap between science and religion," he said, "and this story may be the catapult to do just that!"

12

STEM CELL PIONEERS, ROMAN AND HANS

Alabama and California
2001–2011

It was June 2011, and TJ and I felt the pieces of our book project were finally coming together. Geron had just reported that the first three GRNOPC1 patients were doing well and had suffered no serious side effects from the stem cell injection. I was busy working with our new literary agent, Mac, reaching out to as many patient advocates and research organizations as possible to help establish the bona fides of our proposal to potential publishers. TJ had two new goals he was working on: getting better and stronger, both physically and emotionally.

Since January, when his day program at the Shepherd Center came to an end, TJ had hoped to continue his rehabilitation at Beyond Therapy. Initiated in 2005, Beyond Therapy was yet another of Shepherd's boundary-pushing programs. With facilities in Atlanta, Georgia, and in Franklin, Tennessee, this rigorous program continually operated at full capacity—between thirty and thirty-five clients, each of whom received some twelve to fifteen hours of physical therapy each week. Yet with a perpetual waiting list fifty names long, TJ knew it would be some time before getting in.

It was during his follow-up appointment at Shepherd Center in May that he learned a spot had opened at Beyond Therapy's clinic in

Franklin. Though it was seven hours away from his family in Chatom, TJ knew he had potential to make more progress and wanted very much to keep going. His therapy began from the minute he arrived. In addition to physical therapy (PT) and occupational therapy (OT), he worked with specialists on strength-building and core exercises to help those muscles below the level of his injury recover and possibly demonstrate voluntary motor activity.

Going to therapy week after week, TJ learned that teaching his upper body muscles to control his lower extremities was an exhausting ordeal. But he never once gave up. The gradual improvement he made day after day is what made it all worthwhile—little things like pedaling a bicycle for a few seconds on his own, made TJ push harder the next day. A huge milestone for TJ at Beyond Therapy was the day he was able to crawl on the floor—with quite a bit of assistance, true, but he was moving forward. TJ felt silly cheering aloud to his new friends and therapists, but he was so excited to move forward without the use of his wheelchair.

That same week, I received a Twitter notification from Roman Reed, a patient advocate and legend in the stem cell community, who had himself been paralyzed since 1994. Roman retweeted my direct post to him regarding my interest in interviewing Dr. Hans Keirstead.

I felt I had indeed been blessed again in my effort to help TJ share his story, which needed to include Dr. Hans Keirstead's perspective and involvement in the Geron trial. I swear I did a happy dance around our kitchen before I replied with this:

> RT Thnx @spinalcordcure! #TJAtchison & I R very interested N speaking w/ #HansKeirstead. http://bit.ly/kmU9du #amwriting #TheHumanCandidate @toryminus

I had purposely included a link in my tweet to Roman from his article "Fragile Steps," which just appeared in the current issue of *MIT Technology Review*. I attached the link because I wanted to assure Roman that I had done my research and understood his unique relationship with Dr. Keirstead. Just like his father Don Reed, who wrote for the *Huffington Post*, Roman was an exceptional writer. In that article, Roman explained his first meeting with Dr. Keirstead and his connection to the Geron trials:

> On March 1, 2002, Hans Keirstead handed me the future of medicine. It was a white laboratory rat, and holding it made me feel an odd mixture of

awe, jealousy, and pure joy. It had once been paralyzed, like me. But the rat walked again.

That rat had been given a product derived from human embryonic stem cells—a product that I had played my own role in creating. A California law, the Roman Reed Spinal Cord Injury Act of 1999, had provided Keirstead's initial seed funding. Perhaps never has $92,000 been so wisely spent! The pharmaceutical company Geron acquired the rights to the process and fought its way past many obstacles and hurdles before gaining U.S. Food and Drug Administration approval for human trials. On May 4, 2011, the California Institute for Regenerative Medicine lent Geron $25 million to help with the costs.

These important and required safety tests are hugely expensive. But this first-of-a-kind treatment could transform the lives of many people. Paralysis resulting from spinal cord injury is a devastating condition that currently affects just under 1.3 million Americans. When the various other forms of paralysis are taken into account, 5.6 million Americans have a stake in the outcome.

The Geron trials will not immediately help folks who, like me, have been paralyzed for a while. These first trials are studying the newly injured. But when it comes to paralysis, what helps anyone helps everyone. These trials are creating and codifying a process that can now be used to test other treatments derived from embryonic stem cells—treatments for diabetes, blindness, and more.

These trials could show that we can actually cure the most disabling conditions instead of just maintaining people, often in misery. There are gains for the rest of society, too. Chronic illnesses account for 84 percent of total U.S. health spending, according to the Robert Wood Johnson Foundation. Regenerative medicine like that pioneered in the current trial offers the possibility of cutting those costs and bringing huge gains to the biomedical industry and the whole economy.

Unfortunately, the funding that made this research possible is now endangered. The future of the California Institute for Regenerative Medicine is threatened by the state's ongoing budget crisis. Meanwhile, funding for the Roman Reed Act recently expired, and I am currently campaigning to renew it. The Geron trial is a great start for this field, but we can't let future research with similar potential die on the vine for lack of support.

What Roman's article didn't discuss was the chain of unlikely events that had turned a one-time college football player into a respected and effective patient advocate for those living with spinal cord paralysis. On September 10, 1994, Roman Reed was paralyzed while playing football for Chabot College in Hayward, California. After making nineteen solo tackles, Roman, severely dehydrated and exhausted from playing the entire game, went down for one more tackle. There was a hideous sound, like an axe handle breaking, audible even above the surf-roar of shoulder pads colliding.

The other athletes got up from the pile of bodies and walked away. Roman did not. His neck was broken; he was paralyzed from the shoulders down. Unable to move anything but his right thumb, he gave the crowd a thumbs-up, letting everyone know he was going to be okay. But unfortunately, confirmation of paralysis from a broken neck and shattered spinal cord at C-5 and C-6 was determined at a nearby hospital. At the young age of nineteen, Roman was told he would never walk again or father his own children.

After researching articles from Don Reed's blog, I learned that doctors gave Roman no hope of ever returning to a normal lifestyle. But like the middle linebacker he had once been, who would fight his way through a line of blockers to bring down a runner, Roman was determined to physically recover and to help others along the way. Above Roman's hospital bed, he had a sign made: "I CAN, I WILL, I SHALL." And that became his motto going forward. After months of grueling rehabilitation, Roman recovered the use of his arms and learned to drive an adapted van. He went on to graduate from the University of California at Berkeley with a degree in politics—and passed the law in his home state to fight paralysis.

Inspired by Roman's determination, Assemblyman John Dutra authored a medical research bill, the Roman Reed Spinal Cord Injury Research Act of 1999. Over the next ten years, Roman's Law provided $15 million in California for research while attracting an additional $87 million from the National Institutes of Health and other sources—over $100 million in biomedical research for California.

But just as Don Reed said, "every success led to a larger awareness"; Roman realized that "incurable" illness and injury was far bigger than paralysis alone. He was enraged that in the twenty-first century, approximately one hundred million citizens suffered from chronic disease or disability. So when Palo Alto's Robert Klein inspired Proposition 71, the California Stem Cells for Research and Cures Initiative, Roman had to be a part of it. In Don's article "Light a Candle, or Curse the Darkness," he explained that his son was "always a good salesman. Roman would drive his power chair up to strangers on the street, smiling at them—while demanding their signatures of support for California's stem cell program." Don continued, "It is pretty hard to say no to my son! When he was a boy, he would help his sister Desiree sell Girl Scout cookies. People would buy from him, and then give the cookies back, the box unopened—so Roman could sell them again."

With such a determined spirit, Roman became the spokesperson for Prop 71, even featured in an advertisement created by Jerry Zucker, the legendary director of such films as *Ghost* and *Airplane*. Roman's words even became the official slogan for the Prop 71 campaign: "Turning Stem Cells Into Cures!"

Battling for the cure sums up Roman's approach to life: that to solve a problem is better than to complain about it. When the funding ran out for the law named after him, Roman made the four hour commute to Sacramento, meeting with the legislative aides of every member of the state's assembly and senate, again and again. The program was renewed unanimously in 2005, and signed into law by Governor Schwarzenegger. For over fifteen years, Roman dealt with the pain of experiencing life from a wheelchair, but something beautiful had come from his pain, and his unconquerable spirit was soon to transform my life.

The day after I reached out to Roman on Twitter, he sent back a direct message: "Hi Tory, Send me an email address that I can send to Hans. Take care."

I quickly responded with, "Most grateful 4 your help in putting us in contact w/ Hans! (my email provided)" followed by, "Awesomeness, @spinalcordcure! Am hoping for a day when I can say, 'THANK YOU, #RomanReed!' in person:)!"

Since starting my work in documenting TJ's story in November 2010, I had prayed for the opportunity to meet stem cell pioneers like Roman and Hans to ask them about the science behind Geron's clinical trial. *If only I could have an hour to speak with these men*, I would say to myself while doing late-night computer searches for videos or articles about them. And now, it looked like that dream might happen.

What made Roman such an influential patient advocate? It was not because he was disabled and in a wheelchair, but rather because of his dynamic personality and huge presence on social media websites like YouTube, MySpace, Facebook, and especially Twitter. The new media allowed Roman to connect to a wider community of patients, advocates, scientists, politicians, and donors—connections unheard of a decade before. Roman was tireless in his advocacy and widely admired for his integrity and understanding of the science and economic costs behind patient health care. His tenacious spirit shone like a beacon to all who came to know him. In a word: Roman was a rock star.

From those first exchanges, our friendship deepened over several months. Communicating through Twitter was convenient and easy, and the instant response feature allowed us to develop a natural banter. With many of our followers convinced we'd known each other for years instead of a few months, there was plenty of fun and humor shared between us; but we also developed a very strategic and methodical way to convey our message of support for each other and for stem cell research.

Because I was still new to the discussion around the hot-topic issues of stem cell research, Roman protectively made sure I didn't inadvertently cross over into dangerous territory, especially in correspondence with those who stalked our every move—biotech investors, journalists, or human rights groups who followed our posts. Investor chat groups were saturated with discussions of my Twitter and blog posts that mentioned TJ, stem cells, or the Geron trials. Our literary agent, for instance, cautioned that some investors from competitive biotech companies felt that Roman, TJ, and I were manipulating Geron's stock price by posting comments about TJ's progress. This is one example from a mounting stack of emails sent to our literary agent:

> Mr. Mackie,
>
> I have come across a blog by Tory Minus which says she is a client of your agency. In her blog she is stating that her book is about T.J. Atchison who is the first person in an ongoing trial by the Geron Corp. As an investor, I find it disturbing that Tory is painting a picture to the public that some miracle has occurred with this young man and that she plans to release information on April 9th. I have tried to contact Geron and Tory about her claims to no avail. I would like to know if indeed she is misleading the masses in order to sell books. Someone needs to speak up about this issue, because there is a great deal of attention being paid to her blog and tweets in the investment community.

My father kept a close eye on those investor forums, as several constituted a borderline form of harassment and were filled with derogatory comments about both TJ and me.

Roman helpfully guided me away from this negativity by introducing me to his inner circle of friends and supporters in the biotech community, including the top biotech tweeters like Dr. Paul Knoepfler of UC-Davis; author Rebecca Skloot; CNN's medical program director Miriam Falco; and patient advocate Brooke Ellison, among many others. Most important, Roman was working to connect me with those involved with Geron's clinical trial. On August 28, I received an email from UC-Irvine administrative assistant Michelle Goldman, offering to pencil me in for an appointment to meet with Hans. I was thrilled and immediately juggled everything on my calendar—my job, car pools, children's school activities and playdates, and time-crunching writing deadlines—to make myself available.

We set the date for my visit to UC-Irvine for Friday, September 23. I immediately emailed Roman to share the wonderful news. I couldn't imagine coming to California without also trying to meet him. Luckily, this was Roman's only free weekend that entire month, so we agreed to meet halfway between UC-Irvine and his home in northern California. We discussed several locations but determined there was no better place to meet than in Valencia, California, home to Magic Mountain.

Fast-forward two weeks later, I was heading home from work and just about to pick up my youngest daughter at Spot for Tots Preschool—the center that TJ's mother Anita had expanded from a small day-care to a state-certified program, and where she served as the director—when I received a text from Dr. Keirstead's assistant that he had an opening in his schedule that evening if I was interested in a quick phone chat. I excitedly wheeled my Suburban into the preschool parking lot and ran inside to tell Anita the wonderful news. It was moments like this, seeing the joy on her face that smiled right back at mine, that fueled my efforts and made me work even harder to complete "The Human Candidate."

Courtney and I made it home in plenty of time for me to wrap up homework with the older children and cook them dinner. With just half an hour remaining before my call with Dr. Keirstead, I asked my sister Tera if she could take the children to Wednesday night church service, so my first conversation with Keirstead would be undisturbed. Tera, along with our entire family, was just as anxious as I to get this story out there. They shared in my vision that this book would encourage others in our small community, and across the Bible Belt region, to support stem cell research. We were hopeful this book would cause a ripple effect of support across the nation and the world.

At six o'clock, she hurried my kids out the kitchen door and left me sitting at the table with a few minutes to collect my thoughts before the phone rang. Because the West Coast was two hours behind my central time zone, Dr Keirstead would be calling from his office, his day filled with purpose and significance, and still unfinished. Staring at my watch, I rolled a pen around on the table and waited.

At 6:15 p.m. (CST), my phone lit up with a 949 area code on the screen, and I knew it was Hans. My heart skipped several beats, and my hands shook. I had a list of questions in front of me, I was well prepared, but as I stood up from the table I nearly dropped my phone in nervousness. I didn't know if I should jump straight into my questions or make small talk for the first few minutes. After the third ring, I caught a glimpse of myself in the kitchen window and thought to myself, *Pull yourself together, Tory!* As someone once quipped, the doors of opportunity are marked "Push" and "Pull," and this one was surely a once-in-a-lifetime chance. *Don't miss it!*

I swallowed hard and answered. After a quick and hesitant hello from my end, it was a wonderful relief to hear Dr. Keirstead's immediate enthusiasm, "Hello, Tory! Thank you so much for being in touch and for taking on this incredible challenge." My fears scooted permanently away.

For the next forty-five minutes, we discussed his research and his commitment to helping others. I found Dr. Keirstead to be kind, modest, and down-to-earth, and he made me feel comfortable enough to draw him out about his upbringing, his personal and professional struggles, and about the countless rejections for his research idea that eventually led to the Geron trials. And he insisted I call him Hans. The friendship and loyalty he and Roman felt for one another had opened a wide door for this story, for which I was very humbled.

With time left for only one more question, I asked Hans to describe his greatest accomplishment, whether personal or professional. He chuckled softly and replied, "It's difficult to rank accomplishments, because I believe they are gifts that come at the right time and right place in a person's life. But I'd have to say that in 2002, when I gained a great friend and brother in Roman, I also gained support and funding for my research. Whatever I've accomplished must in part be credited to him. Roman was the first person to take my research seriously. Without a doubt I am where I am because Roman believed in me as a friend and researcher."

Hans had earned and deserved every bit of success that had come his way, but he was exactly right. From the moment Roman held that treated rat named Fighter in his hands at UC-Irvine, he was both in awe and jealousy of the animal. Roman felt the animal's formerly paralyzed legs pushing strong against his hands, trying to get away from his grasp. Her coat was full and healthy, meaning she had no pain. Roman knew that here was the tangible realization of a seemingly impossible dream: to cure paralysis.

Roman returned to his Fremont, California, home and explained to his foundation's scientific grant review committee that the animal walked because of Hans, whose brilliance was matched only by his courage and determination. Other research foundations in the area had denied Hans funding, claiming this rat experiment was "too far reaching." Roman was convinced that money from his law—the Roman Reed Research Act—being channeled into his foundation should award Hans direct funding to further test the concept and provide validity (proof) that this pioneering research could cure paralysis.

Indeed, Roman's and Hans's paths had crossed for an important reason, one that could change the lives of millions of people living with disease and injury. I felt so honored that my path had now crossed with theirs, and that I would soon have an opportunity to meet them both. Just before my departure, Roman emailed a press release from Stanford University Medical Center, announcing a fourth participant had enrolled in Geron's clinical trial.

This new unidentified patient was treated on September 17 at the Rehabilitation Trauma Center at Santa Clara Valley Medical Center with cells prepared for injection at Stanford University School of Medicine. Stanford neurosurgeon Gary Steinberg implanted the cells. Three other patients had previously received the surgically delivered cells: two at the Shepherd Center in Atlanta, beginning with TJ in October of 2010, and one at Northwestern University Hospital of Chicago in May 2011. This new patient was the first person to receive the therapy west of the Mississippi.

Dr. Steinberg spoke about his excitement of participating in this landmark clinical trial, and how it signified a major advance in the effort to one day restore function for patients with stroke and spinal cord injury and for patients with Parkinson's disease and other devastating neurologic disorders.

This exciting news arrived with fortuitous timing and created great momentum going into my trip to the West Coast. On September 22, with my itinerary folder in hand and resource books tucked away in my carry-on bag, I departed Mobile Regional Airport en route to Irvine, California, to meet and interview Hans and Roman. As my plane ascended into a beautiful sunset, I thanked God for allowing things to fall into place for TJ and his story.

The next day, I pulled into a parking lot off of Health Sciences Road and sat for a moment to take in the lovely campus of UC-Irvine. The hilly grasslands, tranquil gardens, and infinity fountains were exactly what I needed to help quiet my nerves and prepare me for the meeting with Hans. With TJ now back home, in nursing school full-time and preparing for an exam, he couldn't make the trip, so I packed a special gift from us both to deliver to Hans, a signed "Pray-for-TJ" shirt, along with a University of Alabama football jersey.

I arrived early at the magnificent, state-of-the-art Sue and Bill Gross Research Center for my one o'clock appointment. After a quick check-in with the receptionist, I paced around the lobby and read a timeline encased along the wall that provided the history of this remarkable research facility. I asked the receptionist if cameras were allowed, and she answered, "Absolutely, just not inside the laboratory."

I snapped as many photos as I could until a man's voice called my name from above. I looked up and saw Hans waving from a balcony that overlooked the lobby. He was movie-star handsome, dressed casually in a dark fitted T-shirt with his brown hair streaked with golden highlights. I grabbed my bags and rushed up a flight of stairs to join him. My heart was racing as we walked down the hallway toward his laboratory. The walls decorated with large photos of stem cells reminded me that the man to my left was perhaps the most brilliant man I had ever met.

For the next two unforgettable hours, we toured the research lab where Hans further explained the science behind his invention, translating that complex process and terminology into simple, understandable information. Seeing the sophisticated microscopes and lab equipment that he had used during the discovery of his paralysis breakthrough, along with glancing inside the "clean room" where his stem cells were stored, I gained a better understanding of the time and effort that had gone into Hans's groundbreaking research.

Following my visit, I drove two hours north of Irvine to Magic Mountain. Roman and I decided it would be fun to meet at the home of Six Flags in Valencia. And because Roman was a diehard sports fan, I felt he would appreciate my appropriately colored houndstooth dress, to represent the spirit of my home state's National College Football Championship team, the Alabama Crimson Tide.

Through a thinning crowd at the entrance lines, I spotted Roman sitting in a burgundy caravan parked along the curb and ran toward him. His long, massive arm extended high above the driver's side window, waving cheerfully until I reached him. He was dressed impeccably in black slacks and a crisp lavender shirt. Roman's brown wavy hair was tucked behind his ears, and his blue eyes were strong and unwavering. We drove over rugged bare hills and past rocky walls to a quaint restaurant away from the amusement park and settled in for our interview.

Roman and I spent over three hours talking about everything from religion to our favorite television shows. And while there was no topic off limits, we were most interested in discussing the torturously slow operation of FDA clinical trials. We dove straight into the barriers of research like seagulls into water, and were in agreement that more should be done to speed the process of bringing a new drug or treatment to patients.

I was thrilled to have found a new friend and a partner for research cures. I asked Roman if he would consider visiting Alabama before the Thanksgiving holiday. I wanted him to meet TJ, but I also had an idea that I began to describe while we drove for ice cream at Baskin-Robbins, an idea that might bring stem cell research into uncharted territory and that would involve introducing him to my close family friend, Senator Marc Keahey. In fact, I had already reached out to Marc and been encouraged by his early response. Roman was immediately interested and said he would do his best to plan a trip as soon as possible.

Before we said our good-byes for the evening, I took out my cell phone and dialed TJ's number. After several rings TJ answered, and I told him that I had someone very special that I wanted to introduce him to. I passed my cell to Roman and, against a sinking sun that lit the earth's edge like creation itself, tears filled my eyes as I listened to Roman and TJ converse. As I knew they would, the two hit if off immediately. They talked, of course, of Alabama beating Arkansas. With everything they had each shared and surmounted, their common ground was this most natural and human of topics. Perfect.

But there was something else. Tears escaped from my eyes as I realized that today was both the eve of what would have been Christopher Reeve's fifty-ninth birthday and the one-year anniversary of TJ's automobile accident. Roman and I looked over our shoulders and noticed a beautiful tower from the amusement park—the Superman: The Escape ride loomed in the distance. I couldn't think of a more meaningful way to end this weekend I'd never forget with Roman and Hans, a weekend that would, in time, change our lives.

13

CASANOVA'S RENDEZVOUS

Alabama and California
September through December, 2011

I was at the John Wayne Airport in Orange County, the last passenger in a long line to board the plane at the American Airlines terminal. Outside it was still dark, but thank goodness the sun would rise before my flight departed. I wasn't a frequent flyer, and the few times I had flown in darkness were not good experiences when my flights had unluckily encountered rough turbulence.

The boarding line had now come to a complete standstill, and I was struggling with my laptop and shoulder bag, while talking to my mom on my cell. I was very tired, as always from my life of perpetual multitasking, but now, after the excitement of the last forty-eight hours, I was finally allowing exhaustion to be felt. In my other hand was a venti coffee, which I hoped would kick in before takeoff. We boarded at 7:45 a.m., and to push me through the half-hour wait time on the tarmac, I took out a notepad and pen and brainstormed ideas of how to get Roman to Alabama to meet my good friend Senator Marc Keahey.

Roman, a football player at heart, a patient advocate by calling, and a political leader by choice, had spent over a decade of his life in a wheelchair, advocating on Capitol Hill for human clinical trials involving embryonic stem cell research to begin. Without a doubt, I knew he was the perfect person to mentor TJ to become a rising patient advocate as well. But then there was my lightbulb moment. I wanted Roman's help for Marc to pass a law structured similarly to "Roman's Law" to provide funding for stem cell research in the Deep South. Yes. It. Could. I just had to find a way to connect these three amazing men before the Alabama legislative session reconvened in January 2012. It would become my top priority.

After an eight-hour journey, including two layovers and a broken strap on my computer bag, I landed in Mobile with a seventy-mile drive still ahead of me. But there was not enough caffeine in the world to compete with the adrenaline rush I felt after having called Roman a dozen times from the airport. The ideas bounced around in my head for the ways we might create an Alabama law bearing TJ's name that would raise awareness and funding for stem cell research in our state. Roman was 100 percent on board, which was crucial to our potential success.

A week later, we had set a meeting for the Veterans Day holiday. Roman would travel to Alabama for a three-day visit with TJ and his family, and to meet Marc. As the time approached, Roman emailed a list of United State senators he knew we could collaborate with if Marc needed that kind of national support. Roman's rich list of relationships and personal contacts enlisted in the cause of stem cell therapy drew from the biotech and political elite around the globe.

Marc was a respected political figure in Clarke County, Alabama, the father of three young children. He was a conservative Southern Baptist and an ardent pro-life supporter. We had spoken many times over the phone about the controversial issue of embryonic stem cell research and the clinical trial in which TJ had participated. He agreed that abandoned embryos from fertility clinics should be available for research, but still had many questions about the process and wanted to know more about the opposition surrounding this research.

Wanting Marc to be as prepared as possible for our upcoming meeting, I emailed a brief overview to him of hESC research, hoping the merit and truth to this technology would outweigh any ethical issues he might have. I was in fact extremely nervous about pressing "send" on this email. But something deep inside told me that Marc would see past the word "embryo" to consider squarely—with real facts and information—past emotion, to look to the science itself, and the fairness of offering a cure to millions living with injury and disease.

I explained that human embryonic stem (ES) cells were unique in medical research for two reasons. First, they alone were totipotent, meaning they could form into any cell or tissue type in the adult body. In addition to forming any cell type, they were unique in their ability to self-assemble into complex multicellular tissues such as intestine or full thickness skin or kidney tissue, and so on. Second was the ease with which they could be purposefully modified in a precise manner that would allow their use in many hundreds of possible clinical applications. And I described how researchers from around the globe were aggressively pursuing lines that could lead to revolutionary therapies for such devastating human ailments as cancer, Lou Gehrig's and Parkinson's diseases, diabetes, heart disease, and, of course, paralysis.

Funding ES cell research would accelerate the delivery of novel therapeutics to afflicted people—people just like twenty-one-year-old TJ Atchison of Chatom, Alabama. Now came the hard part: countering the objections that would surely be raised to this research. Most compelling among these was that the embryo used in this research was a human life and destroying it was the same as abortion or murder of the unborn.

I explained my position in this argument: A preimplantation embryo is not a human life, I wrote, but cells in a petri dish. This cluster of cells is destined to die unless it implants in the uterus to form a pregnancy. Indeed, it is estimated that 50 to 80 percent of these preimplantation embryos naturally formed in a woman's body never implant and therefore die. A human life, as opposed to simply cellular life, begins, at the earliest, at or around day fourteen of human development, around the time the preimplantation embryo attaches to the uterine wall in the mother. Prior to day fourteen, the preimplantation embryo has no body cells of any kind. The embryo is not individualized. It can still in fact become one or two or even more individuals.

I concluded my email by adding my voice to those who believe that human embryonic stem cell technology offers novel pathways to develop lifesaving therapies that will impact the lives of millions suffering from diseases such as Parkinson's disease, diabetes, arthritis, heart disease, kidney failure, spinal cord injury, liver failure, skin burns, and blood cancers, to name only a few.

Until TJ Atchison became the first recipient of human embryonic stem cells, the public noise surrounding stem cells had been dominated by voices claiming that embryo protection is "the" Christian position. But now, however, TJ, a Southern Baptist, had put a face on the potential for human embryonic stem cell therapy, and with that, many—many good, decent and thoroughgoing Christians—were beginning to rethink their positions. I explained *this* was my main goal in writing TJ's story: I want the world to know that people of faith could and should support stem cell research.

Marc emailed me back, asking to meet in person as soon as possible. I could sense in his excitement that he, too, was completely on board. Our first official meeting about the project would take place on Wednesday, September 28, 2011, just three days after returning from my visit with Roman and Hans on the West Coast.

In a corner booth at the Lil' Touch of Cajun Grill in Jackson, Alabama, Marc and I sat across from each other and went through his list of questions. He wanted to review all the ethical issues involved and to understand them thoroughly before he would take a stance either way. Basics first, we discussed the fertilization process of sperm and egg and drew diagrams to help distinguish between ovulation, fertilization, and conception. His greatest concern was very natural, that the headlines would blast him for endorsing human cloning and for supporting a controversial research. This was, after all, small-town Alabama. We knew there would be rough waters ahead, but Marc believed in the mission and was courageously willing to lend his support. After an hour of strategizing our campaign to pass this important legislation, our dinners largely uneaten and our coffee cold, Marc and I determined we needed Roman to meet with our team in Alabama to move the plan forward.

I spoke with TJ during my drive back to the office and updated him on the great news that Marc had agreed to help us pass legislation in Alabama to fund stem cell research in our state. He was just as thrilled as I and couldn't wait to meet Marc and Roman in person.

Then, on Friday, November 11, the dream of bringing stem cell research to the Deep South edged closer to reality as Roman, TJ, Marc, and I gathered for the first time, the men giving one another brotherly handshakes and hugs, and our group chatting together like old friends. My obsession with my tape recorder and note-taking amused Marc and Roman, but I knew this was a historic moment that had to be documented. CNN learned of the meeting by Twitter posts between Roman and me, and even wanted to send a camera crew down from Atlanta to record the gathering, but Marc rightly suggested we hold off media until our launch plan was finalized and in motion.

Over a quiet dinner Marc said, "I've learned that clinical research requires very significant funding to be successful. Our state legislators have had quite a lot of pro-life issues before them, and our constituents don't know much about progressive research. There was a major turnover in the legislature this year. We went from twenty-three out of thirty-five Democratic senators down to twelve. I had been there for only seventeen months, but after our last election, I became the second longest serving Democrat in office. That's an astounding drop. We have a hard road ahead of us, I have to say, because many of these new Republican members are conservatives who took these positions to get support from our voters."

Roman understood Marc's concerns and wanted to know his strategy. "Tell me how you play to sway the pro-lifers to your viewpoint?"

Marc answered, "Well, I intend to educate my colleagues in the legislature and the constituents in our state and stick to the facts. But the particulars of stem cell research are new to me, so I welcome your advice."

"I understand," Roman said as the waitress left after we gave her our orders. "Tell your constituents that stem cell research is a pragmatical solution to real problems. You can be opposed to abortion and human cloning, but not against in vitro fertilization. And so the facts are these: there are over 500,000 embryos discarded annually from fertility clinics that are approved by law to be thrown away in waste dumpsters. Ask your voters this question: Why not use them for scientific research to help get a young man like TJ out of his chair? How a person can defend the other side of this issue is nonsense."

"I agree with you, Roman!" Marc took a long sip from his water glass and turned thoughtfully back to our guest. "Until a person can put himself in your shoes, they should not judge or endorse one viewpoint over another. Just meeting you and TJ makes me see things so differently. It is unacceptable that someone who is able-bodied is throwing stones at you."

"Thank you, Marc. Thank you for getting it." Roman looked at me and smiled. "In California, the way we went after Republican support in our legislature was to address the financial accountability of regenerative medicine. We talked about job opportunities and increasing employment across the state. We all struggle in America with manufacturing jobs.

Thousands of our jobs are going overseas and it's so important that we create jobs in the biotech community and the stem cell field because these are jobs that can't be outsourced from America. And when you look at the medical costs of caring for people like me and TJ, the cost benefit of finding cures versus long-term care is compelling. Last year in 2010, our combined revenue from national corporate and personal income taxes was $1.6 trillion dollars. Yes, trillion with a 'T.'" He paused to let that figure register. "But our medical costs for people who will most benefit from stem cell research," he continued, "was $1.65 trillion. We can't pay for education, infrastructure, security, and defense with this medical burden. We'll go broke as a society if we don't find stem cell cures."

TJ, Marc, and I agreed that this was a key point to remember when we fanned out to begin speaking with our fellow Alabamians.

Roman observed, "If you believe in America's future, then you must believe in stem cell research. And I believe it's a very bright future. Look, the reason I couldn't take the injection like TJ did is because I have scar tissue caused by inflammation. This inflammation is a secondary effect of my football injury, and is the most destructive part because it blocks the connection from my brain to my spine and lower extremities. But there is ongoing research to reverse the scar tissue, so the acute injury trial that TJ participated in can one day be opened up to chronically injured people like me. The inventor of TJ's therapy, Hans Keirstead, is an amazing man. I call him the twenty-first century Albert Einstein. He has an idea for a vaccine that may be able to calm down the inflammation in a spinal cord injury. He and his team are also taking this research a step further to treat spinal muscular atrophy [SMA]. Have you or TJ ever heard of SMA?"

Marc nodded his head indicating he was aware of SMA, a disease that affects the control of muscle movement—crawling, walking, sitting up, even breathing and swallowing. TJ answered, "No, I don't know much about it," so Roman attempted to explain.

After a quick swipe of his passcode bar across his cell, Roman showed Marc and TJ a photo of himself in a hospital room holding the hand of a little girl hooked up to a breathing machine.

"This is Miss G, the strongest four-year-old little girl I have ever met. Like most infants [with SMA], Gwendolyn Strong was diagnosed at six months old. SMA is caused by mutations in genes, and involves the loss of motor neurons in the spinal cord and brain stem. Gwendolyn was diagnosed with the most severe type of SMA—type 1, the number one genetic killer of infants. The earlier the age of onset, the greater the impact on motor function. SMA onset in children [types 2 and 3], teens, or adults [type 4] generally correlates with increasingly higher levels of motor function. If you're familiar with the game Tetris, then you know that the more blocks the player builds, the better their score and ranking. This is kind of how amino acids work. If you have 100 units of amino acid A in a row, and 100 units of amino acid B in a row, they all work with two receptors that go out and get one amino acid and bring it back to their row to help build the chain even longer. Unfortunately, if diagnosed with SMA type 1, these babies do not have receptors or the ability to go out and get that one amino acid or building block. Using stem cells, Hans has figured out how to educate that second receptor into tricking that one amino acid into coming back and attaching itself to the building blocks. It's amazing progress and fantastic what Hans has discovered."

As the father of three young children of his own, Marc was immensely disturbed by the prevalence of SMA type 1—sixteen out of every 100,000 babies are born with it—and by its devastating side effects.

Staring at his picture of Gwendolyn, Roman answered, "The progressive weakness and waste of this disease is heartbreaking. The muscles die from the inside out while the brain is unaffected, so that babies and young children living with SMA are aware of their pain and suffering. Just a few weeks ago, on October 26, the Roman Reed Foundation held a fundraising event at the Sue and Bill Gross Stem Cell Research Center to raise money for Hans to start a clinical trial for SMA using hESC. I believe with every fiber in my being that hESC will lead to cures for disease and injury. Every cell in our bodies—our eyes, ears, hair, bones, livers, heart muscles . . . everything came from hESC tissue. So if we can tell the hESC what to become, then it will become that part of the body," he explained as our main courses arrived. "Think of a coding system on the Internet," he continued as we began to eat. "You tell the cells what to become. Codifying is exactly what Hans did for spinal cord injury repair. He told them to become oligodendrocytes (the wrapping around the spinal cord which becomes the myelin sheath), and so they did."

"The things we can cure with these cells will also cure our economy and country," Marc added. "It's a ripple effect. We're losing so much time now because research funding is being cut so drastically. It's a huge problem and this sounds like the perfect solution."

Roman's smile widened now that Marc was seeing the big picture of the fiscal accountability for research. He, too, began to dig in to his dinner.

Marc continued, "We are so very lucky to have Roman visit and to educate us on the progress he and others are making for stem cell research." Then, with his brows furrowed, he said, "I don't know whether constitutionally Alabama can handle bills dealing with stem cell research. I'll need to research this over the weekend. I know that the majority of funding would need to come from federal sources unless we can find wealthy individuals who would rally behind us. Roman, please tell us how your state has been successful in funding billions of dollars for California stem cell research?"

"So we're really blessed to have passed Proposition 71 in 2004, which is an incredible $3 billion California bond program that is staggered over ten years for stem cell research in our state. I'll use my great friend and brilliant researcher Hans Keirstead as an example. Because my father Don Reed and I were instrumental in establishing Proposition 71 and were leading sponsors, we were able to showcase the early success of Hans's hESC research, which as you know led to the Geron trials and to TJ's injection. Through Prop 71, we pushed for education and advocacy. The management team behind Prop 71 invited me to serve as education spokesperson. We were successful in securing private funding first, which was then matched with state and federal funding that recognized California as a national leader in the field. All this was taking place during the George W. Bush presidency, when he limited stem cell research to seventy lines. Only twenty of those lines really worked, and these were based on fetal cells of frogs. But researchers didn't want frog cell parts, so even these twenty lines were no good. Bush set the field back by a decade and almost destroyed any chance for a comeback. Seriously. So California took over, basically because there was no other choice. In 1999, we passed a law bearing my name, the Roman Reed Spinal Cord Research Act, and this provided the first funding in the world for hESC. So my point in saying all of this is that if you can secure private funding, then the federal funding will come."

By now we had been joined for dessert by TJ's mother, my friend Anita, and her husband and a small group of friends and fervent supporters. The conversation continued as Anita asked, "How have you responded to those who accuse you of killing babies with stem cell research?"

"I tell them the truth. Babies are not being killed because these cells *have not* differentiated and therefore are not destined to become life. They are, however, destined for a garbage dump. There are no wombs inside the laboratory. Therefore, there is no life inside the laboratory."

"That's powerful information," Marc added. "Nobody knows these embryos are thrown away. You'd have to be against fertility clinics too if you're against hESC therapy."

We were making great progress and so I now asked Roman, "What would be our first steps to begin a law in Alabama?"

Roman smiled. He knew this would be my single question that evening. "Based on my own law in California, I recommend you pass an initiative that proposes funding for stem cell research in Alabama by getting over 85 percent of all registered voters signatures on a petition. People like initiatives because they often feel these laws are from the heart and champion something important. The initiative should be named in honor of a citizen affected by the cause, like TJ. And you guys can use Facebook and Twitter to help solicit signatures. You're lucky: we passed Roman's Law before there was social media, and could only go door-to-door with our signature lists. Initiatives are the best way to go!"

Scratching his head, Marc said, "Unfortunately, Alabama is not an initiative state, so we can't go the petition route to pass a law here. But the new session begins in January, and I will introduce a bill then into legislation and be the sponsor. We can call it TJ's Law, how does that sound?"

TJ's face filled with happiness. He said, "You mean it? That sounds awesome!"

Roman was excited too. "Marc, that's incredible! It took me two years to find a state senator who would sponsor my law. TJ, you've got a great team behind you, and for Tory to have found you a sponsor so immediately is amazing. I'll help you all the way." He paused as the wait staff cleared the table. "One of the first things I suggest you do is to find out the governor's position on stem cell research. If he supports it, that will be huge for us."

Having served with Governor Robert Bentley (R) in the House of Representatives, Marc shared his take on the gentleman. "He's a former dermatologist, and even though he's a conservative Republican, he's likely to support this bill because of his medical background. He's a middle-of-the-road guy, not a right wing extremist. Hopefully he'll see our perspective."

"Marc this is your bill, the TJ Atchison Spinal Cord Injury Research Act. If you have the governor behind you, that's golden. We had Arnold Schwarzenegger's support when he was California's governor, and I'll be indebted to him forever on that. Once you establish a research fund account, scientists will flock to Alabama. And as Alabama becomes the first red state to fund stem cell research, there will be five to six other states coming to you for support because you will be the only source of funding for the southeast. Cures come from research, and research comes from funds. You'll be the light in the darkness, and my friends and I will help you through the process. Onwards and upwards for cures, and for TJ's Law!"

We cheered, "Hear, hear!"

14

A SCREECHING HALT

Jackson, Alabama
November 2011

I first learned the identity of Geron's fifth patient on November 21, 2011, after stumbling across an article from the *Pleasanton Weekly* on Twitter. The only person I knew who could validate this story was Roman, so I texted him to confirm that Katie Sharify had enrolled as the fifth patient in the trial.

Not only did Roman confirm her identity, he also introduced us via Twitter, and soon she and I were emailing back and forth. Katie granted me a phone interview in which she described the events surrounding her participation in the trial.

Just twenty-three, Katie was returning to Los Angeles from a short visit with her family when the noise of rolling energy drinks on the floor of the passenger side of her vehicle grew louder and louder. So while driving down Interstate 5 with her cruise control set to seventy, Katie removed her seatbelt and leaned over to move the cans. A second later, she lost control of her car and began flipping into the hills. The impact ended up sending her through the back window, ejecting her twenty feet away from the wreckage.

In a matter of seconds, this bright, stunning girl who was saving money to re-enroll at the University of Southern California, now lay unconscious, barely hanging on to life. A passerby who witnessed the horrific accident pulled over to the service lane and called 9-1-1. An hour later, Katie was airlifted to Doctors Medical Center (DMC) in Modesto, where she was treated for head injuries, broken ribs, and a damaged spinal cord. She was given blood transfusions and underwent emergency spinal fusion surgery to repair her broken spine.

Physicians at DMC were aware of Geron's stem cell trial and were on the lookout for spinal cord injury patients who might meet the study's inclusion criteria. After observing Katie for several days in ICU recovery, she was identified as a possible participant. A week later, she was transferred to Santa Clara Valley Medical Center to begin rehabilitation and screening for the Geron clinical trial. Upon Katie's arrival, she was approached by a research team who would use the same unique stem cell injection protocol that TJ had been given, just one year prior.

Katie wasn't certain what a stem cell was, but she feared the reality of being paralyzed for the rest of her life and was therefore open-minded to the new therapy. She wanted to find out as much as she could about stem cells and regenerative medicine, and so she searched online and googled the Geron trial. She also learned about TJ from Bob Stein's *Washington Post* article and from stumbling across my blog at Head in the Clouds. Nothing she read indicated that TJ had experienced any negative side effects from the cells, so she was encouraged that there might be something to this technology.

From the start of her research, Katie understood that embryonic stem cells were controversial and experimental. However, this posed no moral issue for her as she did not share in the belief that life begins at conception. Rather, her reluctance to participate in the trial hinged on two issues: 1) she wanted to make certain the procedure would not hinder her body's natural healing process and 2) there would be no further damage caused to her spinal cord, specifically that she would not lose sensation and injury level beyond her current diagnosis as a complete T3. Losing hand function was now her biggest fear, which could easily happen if she sustained an injury above T1. With the clock ticking for her to make a decision, she sought advice from her family and closest friends, and put her questions to the medical team.

On Monday, November 14, just two days before Katie would need to undergo the surgery, Dr. Steve McKenna, Santa Clara Valley Medical's rehabilitation trauma center chief, assured her that, based on the evidence collected so far, the injection procedure appeared to be safe and should cause neither further harm to her body nor hinder her natural recovery. After talking with Dr. McKenna, she knew this was a really big deal for medical research and that she would be helping millions of others by her participation.

Deep into his explanation of the surgery with Katie, Dr. McKenna was interrupted by a colleague, Dr. James Crew, who urgently called Dr. McKenna to the door. It seemed the center had just received a message that Geron had officially halted its stem cell studies, including the GRNOPC1 study, effective immediately.

Katie didn't understand much of the conversation, but from what she could interpret, she heard that the company sponsoring the trial had decided to halt all stem cell studies including GRNOPC1. The news upset her greatly, but she hoped that because she had already signed the preliminary consent forms and passed the screening process, she could still receive the cells. In that moment, Katie went from being a potential candidate to knowing that, if given the opportunity to participate, she would.

Back home in Alabama, I was sitting at my desk at work finishing up my last to-do's for the day when I received an email notification from my contact at Geron, Anna Krassowska. Anna had been so kind to answer questions about the trial for my research. But now she wrote:

> November 14, 2011
>
> Dear Tory,
>
> I apologize for the formal-sounding note. I am writing to let you know that going forward, Geron will focus on its oncology programs and will not be funding further development of its stem cell programs. As part of this decision, we will close the GRNOPC1 trial for spinal cord injury to further enrollment, and are seeking institutional or corporate partners for all of our stem cell programs.
>
> As discussed in the press release below, by narrowing our focus to oncology, we anticipate having sufficient resources to reach important clinical development milestones occurring over the next 20 months in our oncology programs.
>
> Geron will continue to follow all enrolled patients in the Phase 1 study, accruing data and updating FDA and the medical community on their progress. To dispel any concerns, I want to assure you that the decision was not

> based on any safety signals arising from our GRNOPC1 trial. In this trial, GRNOPC1 has been well tolerated with no serious adverse events.
>
> As I am sure you will appreciate, we need to spend the next several days working with our affected employees. However, I would like to arrange a call with you early next week in order to answer any questions that you may have. Could you please suggest possible days and times that would be convenient for you?
>
> I look forward to talking with you soon,
>
> Anna
> Anna Krassowska, Ph.D.
> Investor and Media Relations, Geron Corporation

After reading Anna's message and the accompanying press release, my heart sank for Dr. Hans Keirstead, TJ, and the other trial participants. I called TJ and Anita, and shared in sadness this most upsetting news. They were understandably frustrated and disappointed that no one from Geron had called to give them a heads-up about this impending setback. They felt the entire stem cell field was now in jeopardy. The only hope I could give them was Anna's promise that Geron would continue to monitor TJ and the other participants, but it did not appear Phase I would be completed unless another company agreed to take over the trial—something that could happen, although it seemed unlikely at this point due to the trial's key scientists and management team no longer being a part of the operations at Geron. The company's press release did not change the importance of TJ's role in medical research moving forward. My greatest concern was what effect it would have on TJ's long-term follow-up care. For this assurance, I would have to wait a week for Anna's call. Quite correctly, Geron would indeed acknowledge their commitment to monitor the five patients for fifteen years.

Fast-forward two days later to November 16: Katie Sharify received the news that she had been grandfathered in to the trial by Geron and would be the fifth and final patient injected with GRNOPC1. Stanford's Dr. Gary Steinberg and Dr. Marco Lee from Valley Medical performed the surgery and considered this final injection of GRNOPC1 to be a total success.

Katie came out of anesthesia knowing that many would question her judgment about participating in the trial while knowing that Geron had halted the study. The choice had been hers to make, and she felt no coercion or pressure from anyone to go ahead or not to. A pessimist before her accident, she felt there was so much to be optimistic about in her future. By participating in the trial, Katie believed she was turning the tragedy of her lost mobility into a huge positive by helping to move science forward and, in the process, hoped she would be helping others, too. Even if the GRNOPC1 trial never resumed, Katie knew she was helping researchers understand more about hESCs. This gave her a sense of purpose that she desperately needed at the time. It made her a stronger person and more appreciative of everything in her life each day. Katie no longer wasted her time, energy, and emotions on the trivial things in life. She now saw the bigger picture.

15

TAKING A STAND

Millry and Mobile, Alabama
November 2011–January 2012

The Geron announcement was a real eye-opener for everyone, but especially for Marc, TJ, and me. We now understood the crucial significance of public funding and wanted to take our stand with Roman to help others benefit from stem cell therapy. We had assembled an excellent, dedicated team and felt certain that we could play a huge part in bringing research dollars to the state, so long as we stayed active and coalesced for the cause.

Roman took the immediate lead by introducing Marc Keahey to his hero, Assemblyman John Dutra of California, who had sponsored the Roman Reed Spinal Cord Injury Research Act in 1999. Below is the introductory email sent to John and Marc on November 14th that officially launched our campaign for TJ's Law in Alabama.

> Dear John,
>
> It is my complete pleasure and more important, impactful for the cause of paralysis research and cure, to introduce you to Alabama Minority Whip Senator Marc Keahey. With the highest praise, he is a kindred spirit of yours.

Our friend will be introducing legislation along the lines of The Roman Reed Spinal Cord Injury Research Act for heroic TJ Atchison, as you know the world's first recipient of Hans's research that was temporarily stopped today because of lack of Geron funding. I have consequently brokered a deal between Big Pharma and Hans to revive and be able to take the crucial research all the way from bench to bedside.

I will be devoting my time and energy to get the TJ Atchison Spinal Cord Injury Research Act signed into Law, and will help coordinate and enact the everyday tasks of getting the voting blocs needed, and letters of constituent support needed (Note—not signatures as in an Initiative process like Prop 71), for persuading legislators to vote in our favor and bypass conservative Pro Life opposition.

John, please offer your incredible guidance to this matter that we did so well more than a decade ago. Wordsmithing is a KEY point to defuse those Representative right-winged, anti-stemcell stance. The legislation we are proposing is the TJ ATCHISON SPINAL CORD INJURY RESEARCH ACT. Where does that name mention anything about controversial stem cells? The science will be decided by an impartial and top scientific advisory board on a transparent, grading acknowledged, NIH process. That is how my law works and we fund tons of other great projects. We have to get TJ's Law passed! There is no program like this in the southeast; we will help TJ make history for a second time!

We can get Representative support by engaging the Chambers of Commerce using these three points:

1) Jobs—We create jobs that cannot be outsourced. From building labs, to student postdoc support, to grants, to top Docs in the World right here in Sweet Home Alabama.
2) Fiscal Responsibility—For every one dollar that my law spent using State funds, four dollars came back in matching out-of-state grants. Out of $14 million given from State funds $74 million came back out-of-state matching grants!
3) Curing the suffering and saving our Country—When $1.6 trillion in combined Corporate & Personal Income Tax revenue is weighted against long term healthcare expenditures of $1.65 trillion for our fellow Americans like TJ and me, it is clear we cannot afford to do nothing. America cannot focus on education, infrastructure, or even defense without going bankrupt unless we bring healthcare costs under control. Our research is a step in that direction!

Bandaids are too expensive and they don't heal the suffering for TJ, Gwendolyn Strong, or the 5.6 Million Paralyzed Americans.

All for Cure-And-Cure for All!
Yours,
Roman

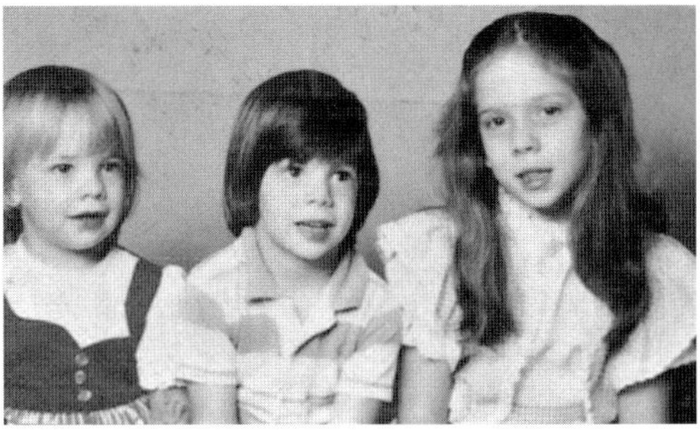

With my brother Brandon and sister Tera, 1979

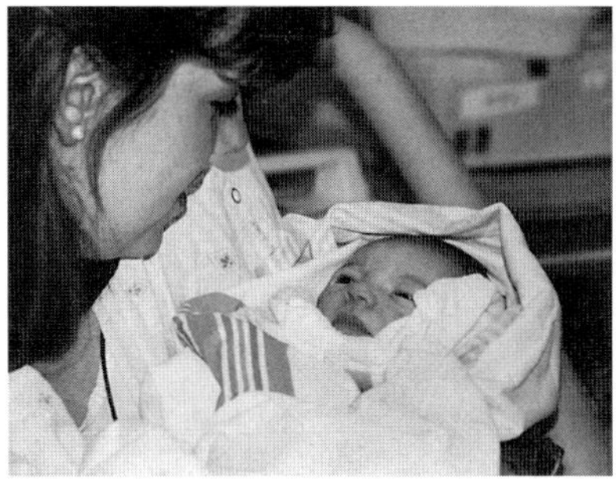

My firstborn, Catie, 2001

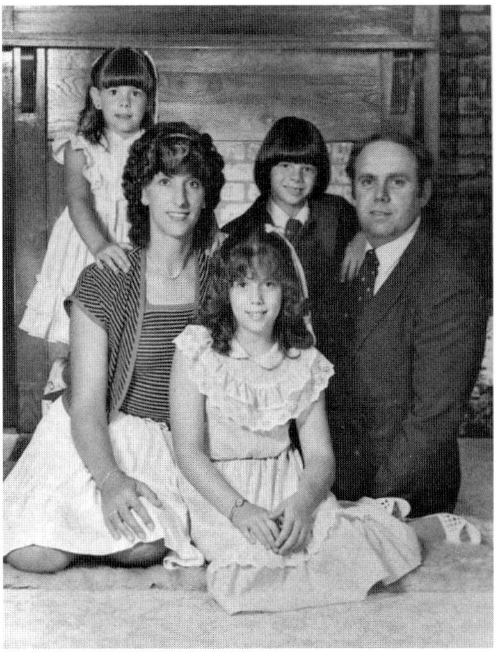

The Armstrong family, 1983
Back row: me
Middle row from left: My mom, Brandon, and my dad
Front row: Tera

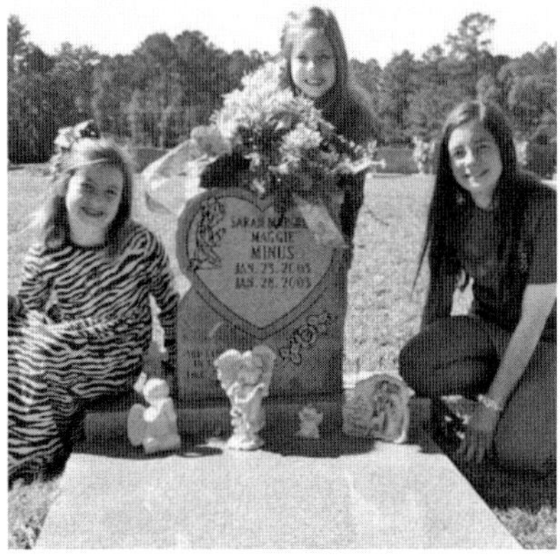

Courtney, Carlie, and Catie visiting their sister Maggie's grave

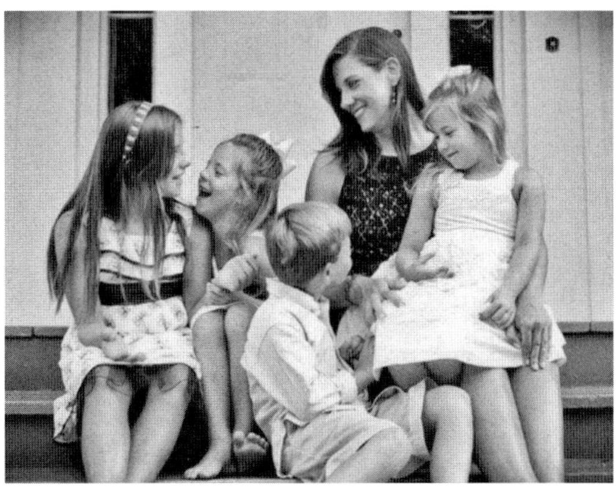

With my four little miracles *(from left)*: Catie, Carlie, Conner, and Courtney

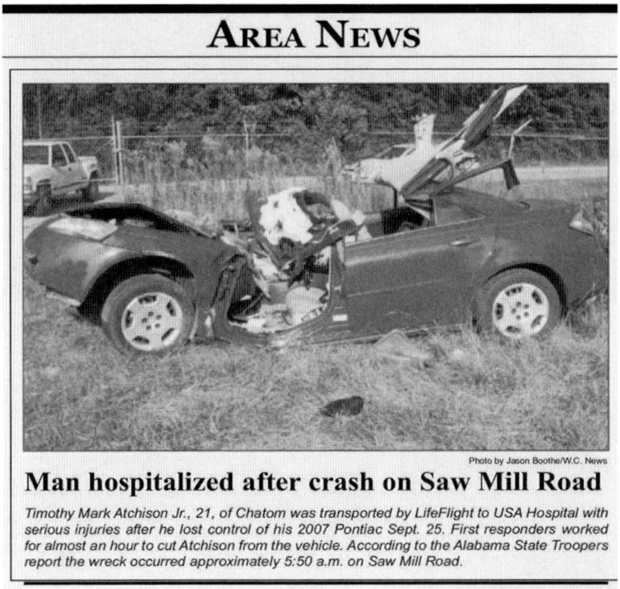

AREA NEWS

Photo by Jason Boothe/W.C. News

Man hospitalized after crash on Saw Mill Road

Timothy Mark Atchison Jr., 21, of Chatom was transported by LifeFlight to USA Hospital with serious injuries after he lost control of his 2007 Pontiac Sept. 25. First responders worked for almost an hour to cut Atchison from the vehicle. According to the Alabama State Troopers report the wreck occurred approximately 5:50 a.m. on Saw Mill Road.

Washington County News write-up about TJ's accident (by Jason Boothe)

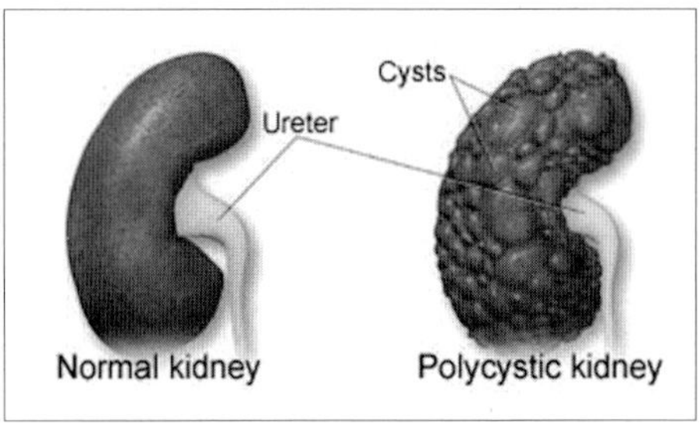

A closer look at Polycystic Kidney Disease (PKD)

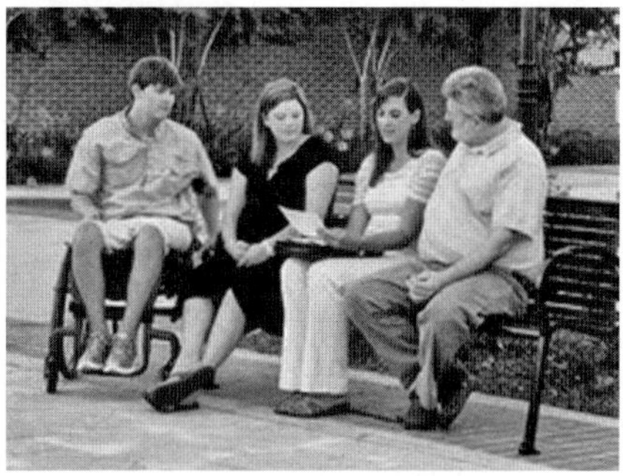

TJ and I interviewing his classmate Mary Lauren Bailey and Professor Joe Farmer at University of South Alabama campus in Mobile

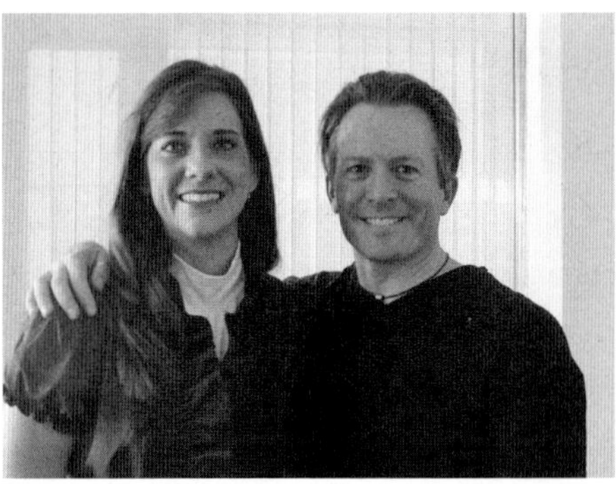

My first meeting with Dr. Hans Keirstead at The Bill and Sue Gross Stem Cell Research Center at UC-Irvine

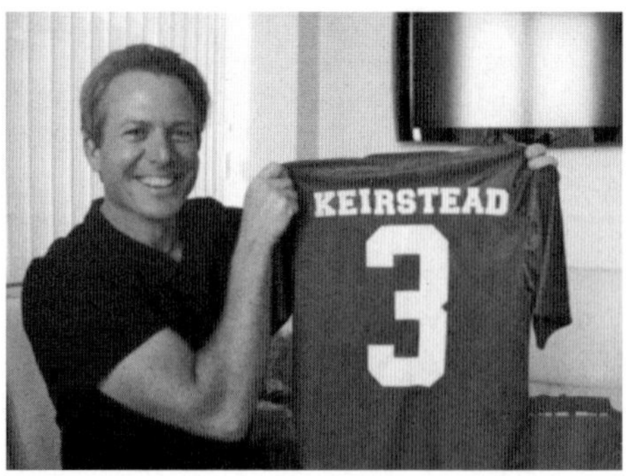

Dr. Keirstead receiving a gift from TJ and me—a University of Alabama football jersey

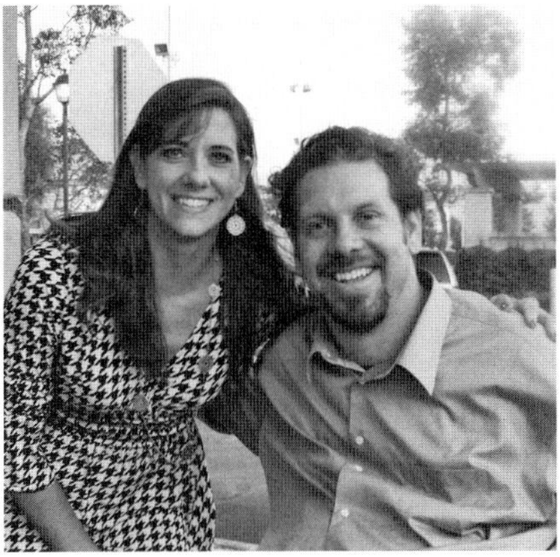

My first meeting with Roman in Valencia, California, home to Magic Mountain

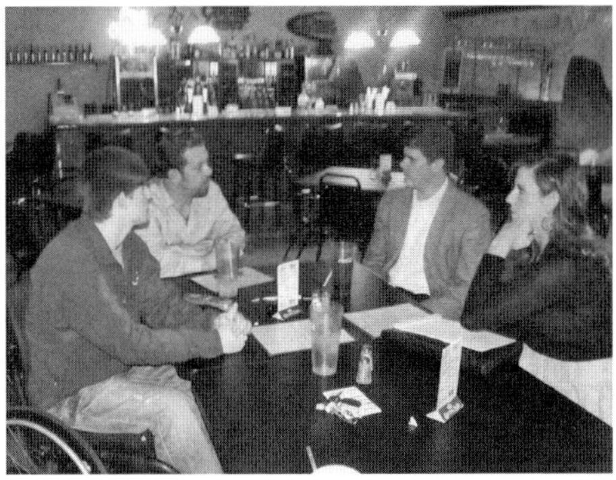

Roman's first visit to Alabama, meeting at Casanova's Rendezvous in Chatom. *From left:* TJ, Roman, Senator Marc Keahey, and me

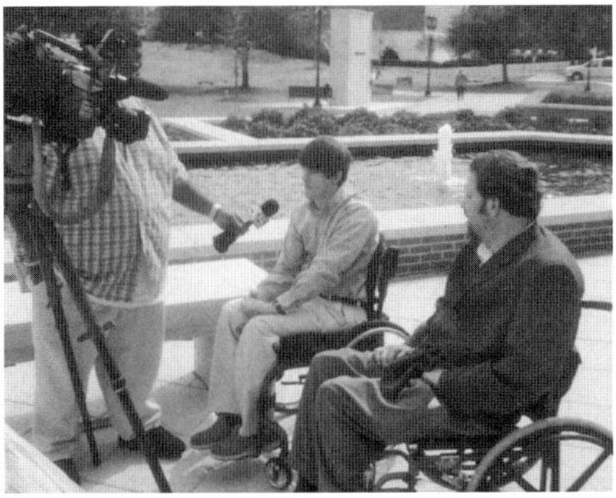

TJ and Roman being interviewed after the press event by local Mobile news station WKRG

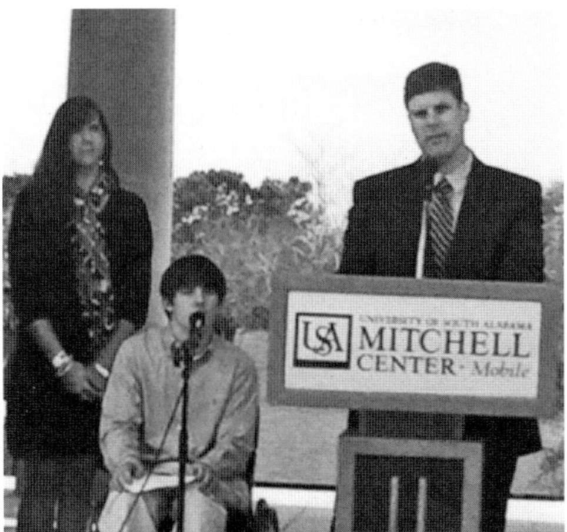

Senator Keahey announces his sponsorship of TJ's Law at a press event at the University of South Alabama campus in Mobile

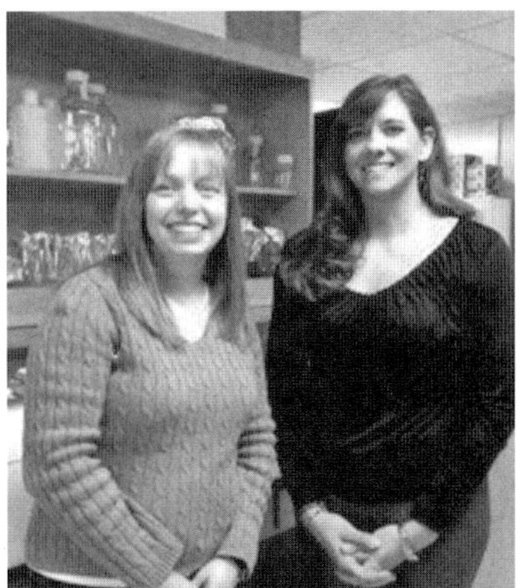

Dr. Candace Floyd giving me a tour of her laboratory at UAB's Spain Rehabilitation Center

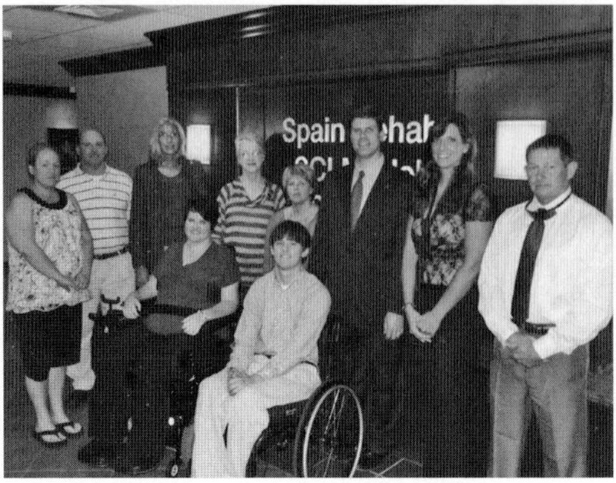

Supporters of "TJ's Law" tour the SRC

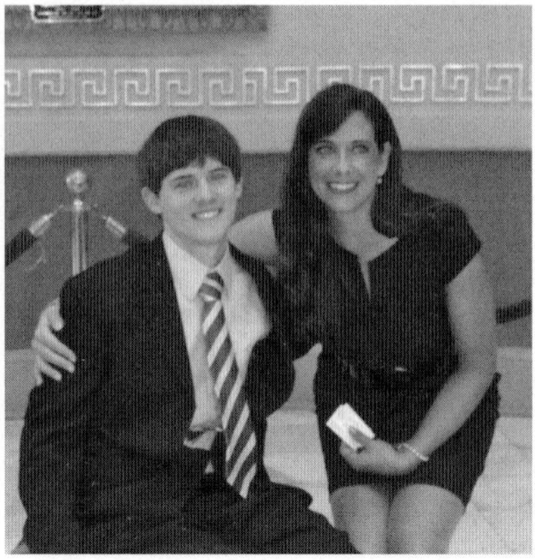

Passing TJ's Law—TJ and I celebrate this victory at the Alabama state capitol in Montgomery

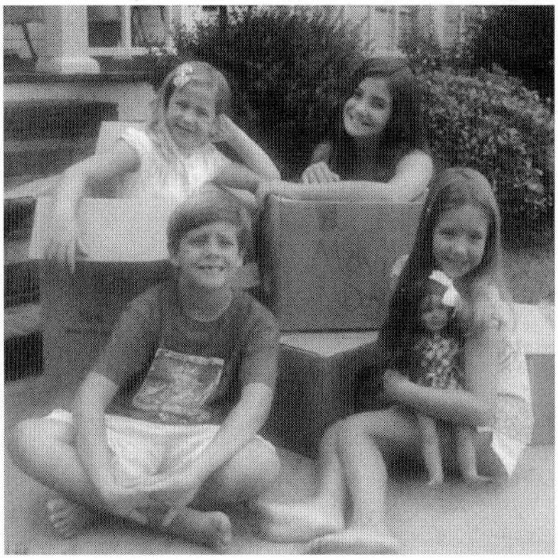

My children pack for our move to Birmingham

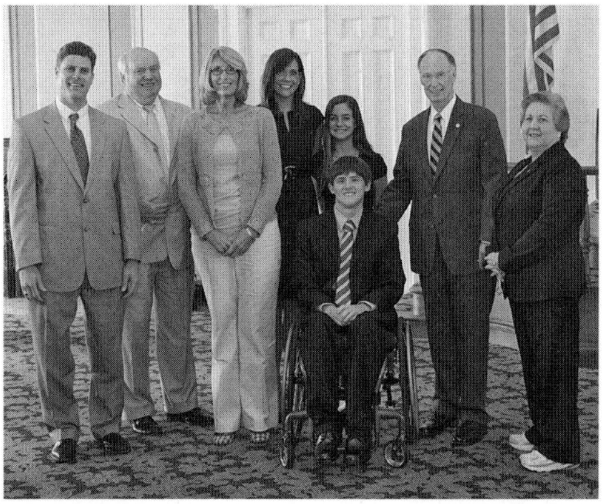

Ceremonial bill signing of "TJ's Law" with Alabama Governor Robert Bentley. *From left:* Senator Keahey, my parents (John and Glenda Armstrong), me, and Catie, TJ, Governor Bentley, and Representative Elaine Beech

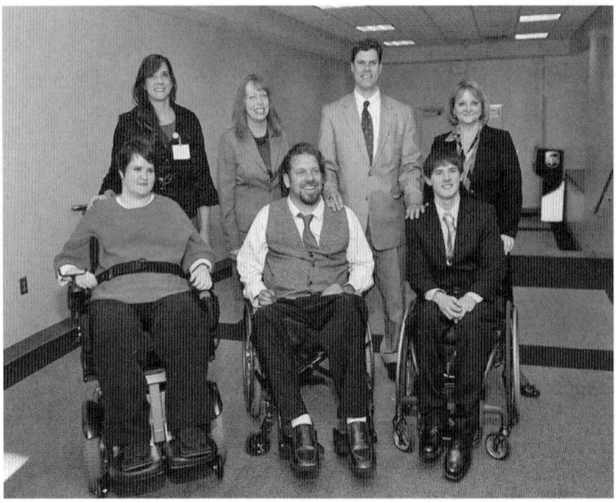

Ribbon cutting ceremony at UAB for the TJ Atchison Spinal Cord Injury Research Program

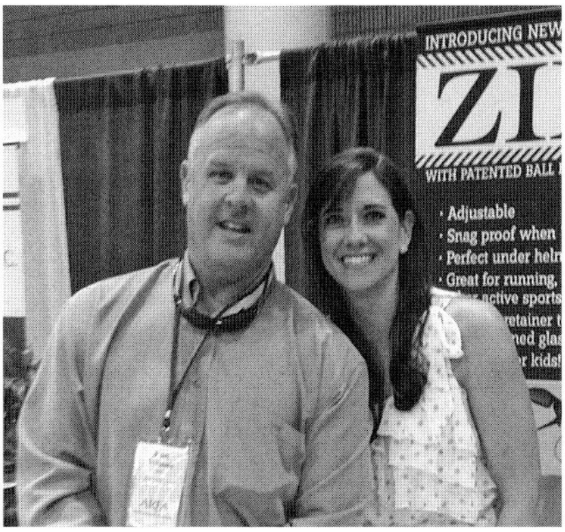

Ron Williams and me during the early days of our courtship

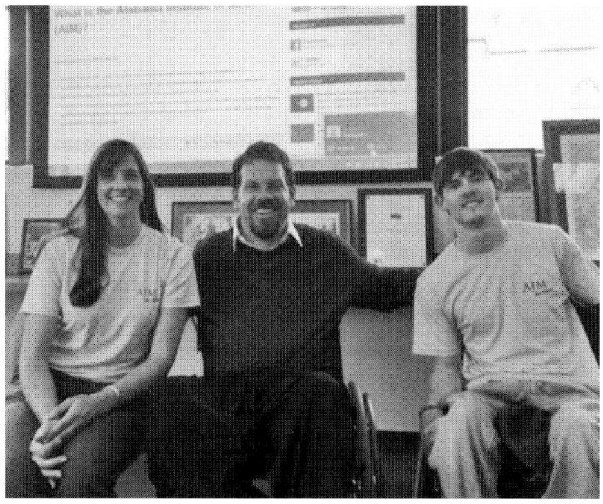

Roman, TJ, and I launching AIM at a Birmingham press event

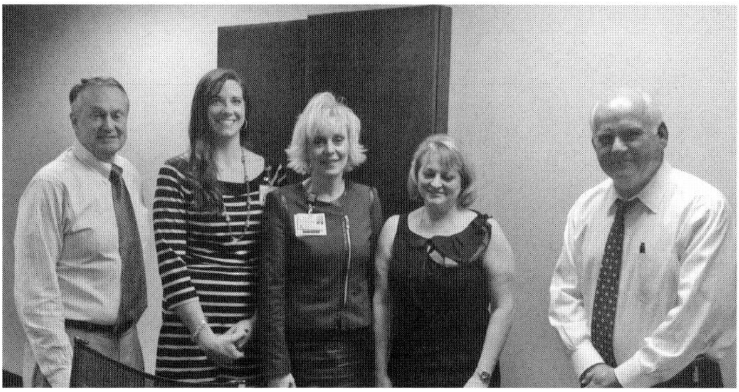

Pitching the new AIM initiative to UAB administrators. *From left:* Dr. Richard Marchase, me, Yvonne Akins, Dr. Amie McLain, and Dr. Ray Watts

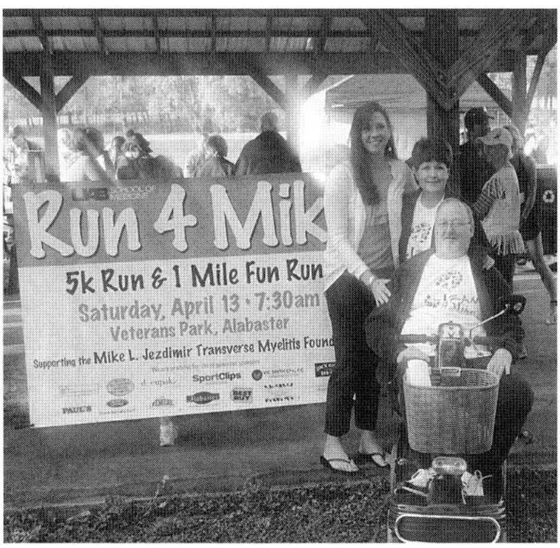

With Louann and Mike Jezdimir at a fundraising event for the Mike Jezdimir Foundation in Alabaster

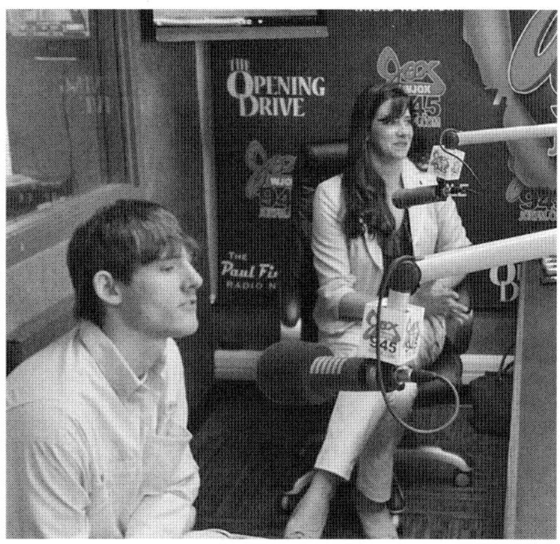

TJ and I promote stem cell research on Birmingham's JOXFM radio station

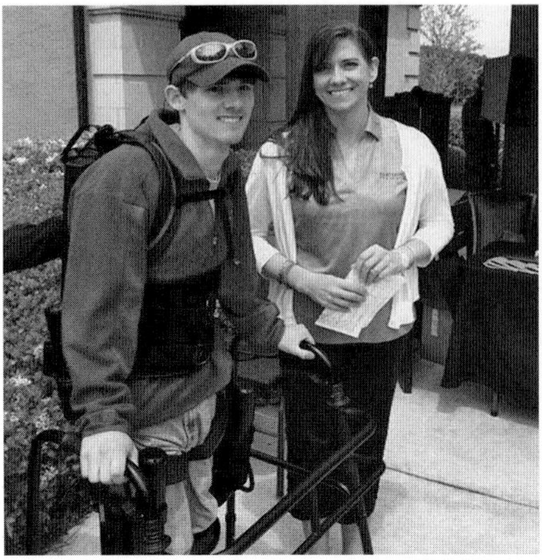

TJ walking in the Eksoskelton suit at the TJ Atchison Golf Tournament (by Fred Powell)

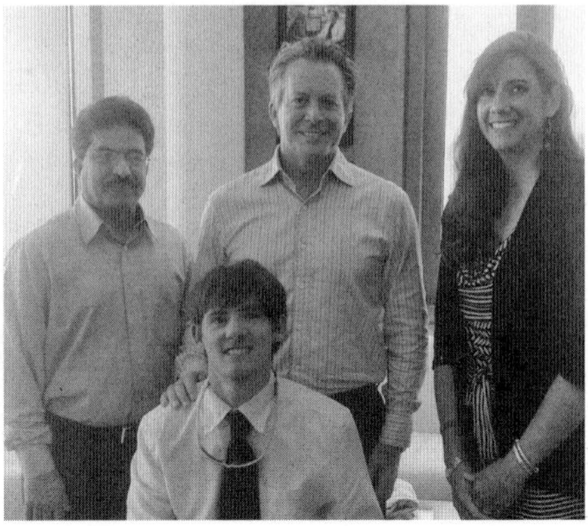

With TJ, Dr. Raj Singh, and Dr. Keirstead at UC-Irvine

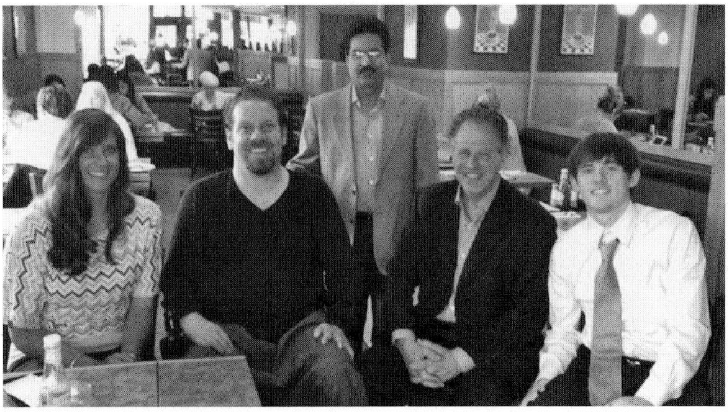

Roman, Dr. Singh, Robert Klein, TJ, and I discuss our new AIM-4-Cure campaign

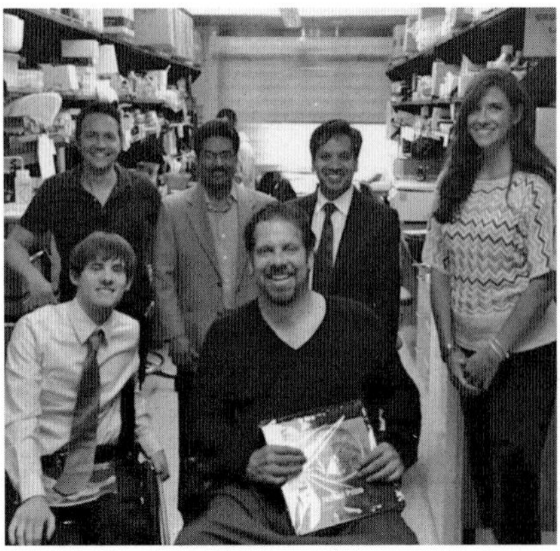

TJ, Roman, Dr. Singh, and I meet with Dr. Deepak Srivastava *(back row standing next to me)* of Gladstone Institute

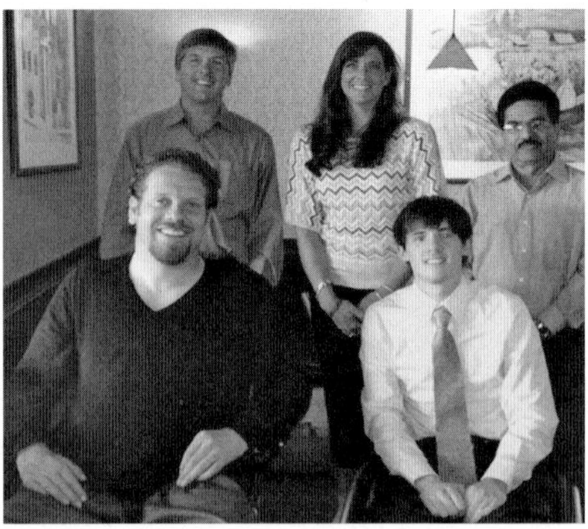

Former Geron medical director Dr. Edward Wirth meets with us during our California visit

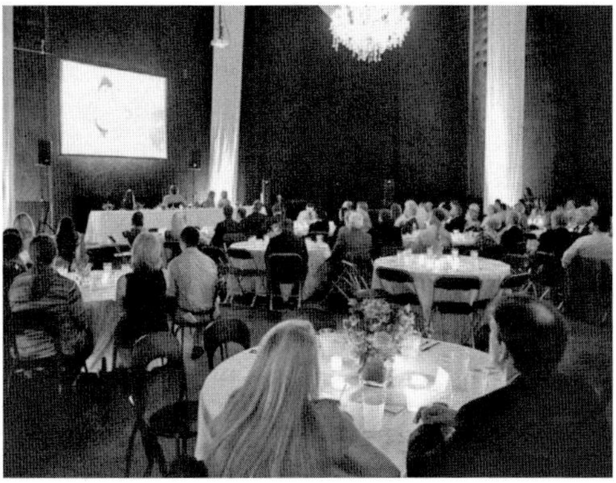

AIM's inaugural Workplay Gala 2013

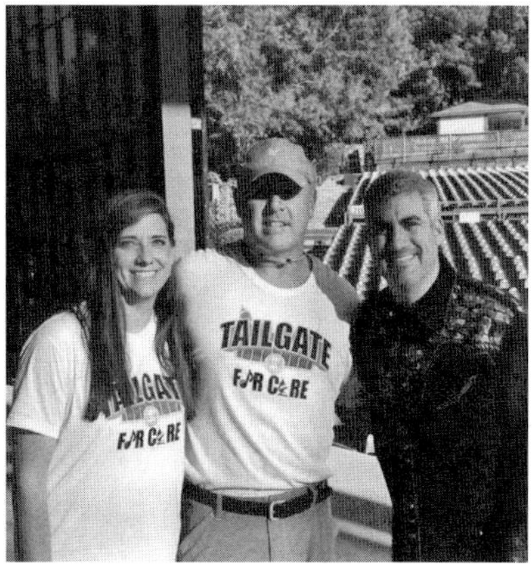

Ron and I with Taylor Hicks before he takes the stage at AIM's Tailgate for Cure concert

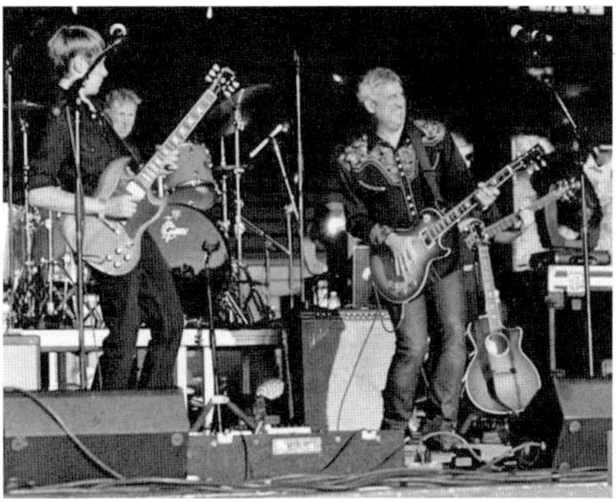

Taylor Hicks giving a great performance

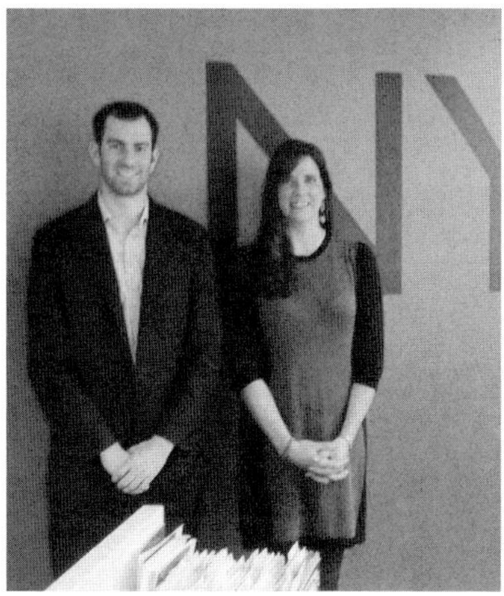

With David McKeon, the New York Stem Cell Foundation chief of staff

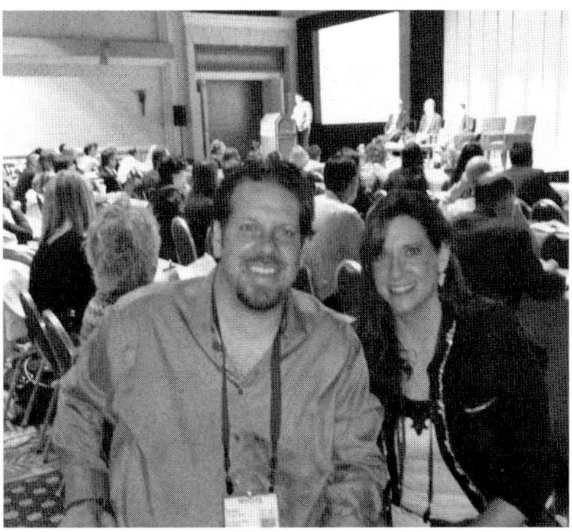

Roman and me during the World Stem Cell Summit in San Diego, December 2013

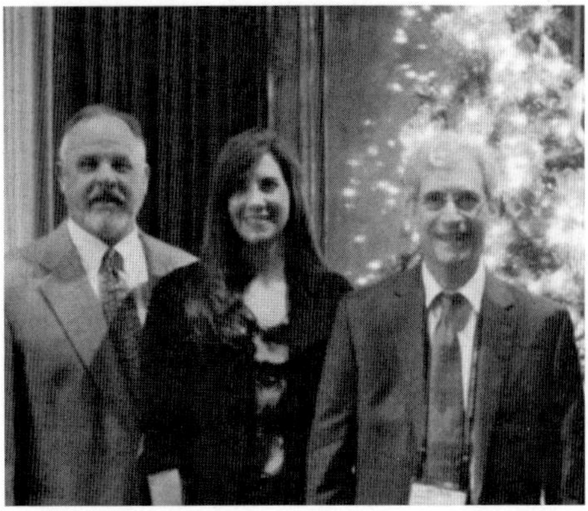

With Ron and Bernie Siegel at the World Stem Cell Summit, December 2013

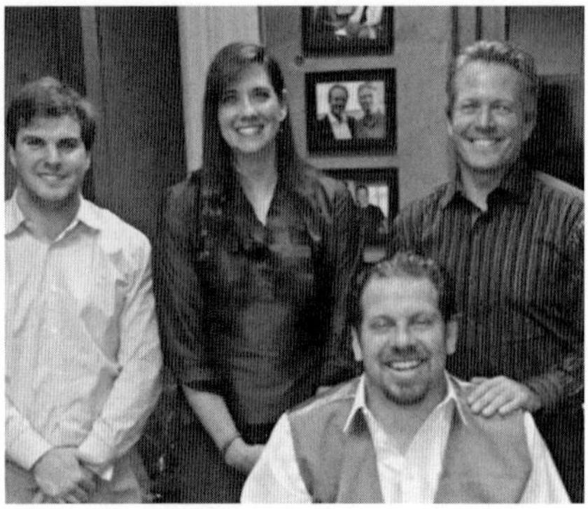

Chris Drummond, Roman, and I discuss a potential collaboration with Dr. Keirstead

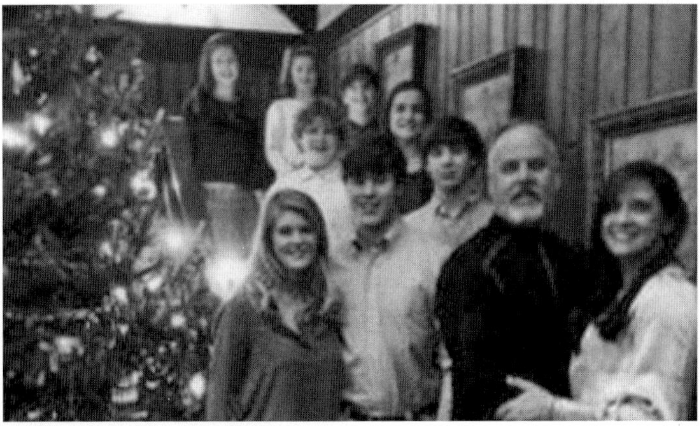

Williams family, Christmas 2013

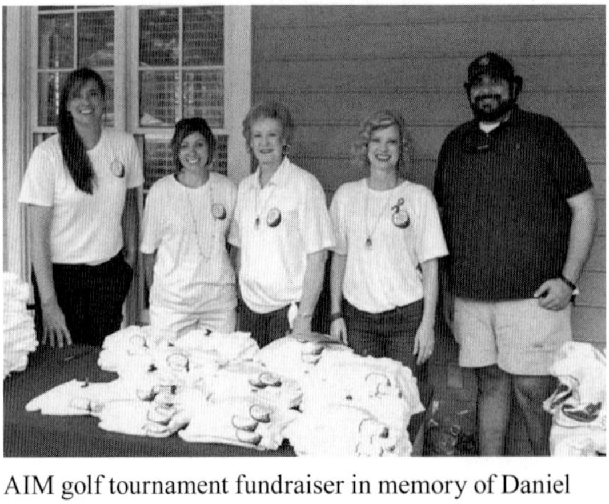

AIM golf tournament fundraiser in memory of Daniel Wayne Robertson, who passed away in October 2013 from complications of transverse myelitis

ALABAMA INSTITUTE
AIM
OF MEDICINE

AIM Logo

Roman sent out dozens of support letters like this to his contacts in both the biotech and political communities across the country. This was his playground, and he knew that if we were going to be successful in Alabama, we had to strike when it was most opportune—when people were finally paying attention to the science headlines and learning about the biotech industry and clinical trials. Most importantly, people were finally understanding the enormous amount of funding needed to bring a new drug therapy to market. We had to take advantage of this news environment and maximize our efforts following the Geron announcement.

One of Roman's contacts was a scientist and friend at the University of Alabama at Birmingham (UAB), Dr. Candace Floyd. Before joining UAB, Candace had been a spinal cord injury researcher at UC-Davis, whose work Roman had twice funded through his program in California. Recruiting her to our team was a stroke of genius, or seemed to be at the time.

We all understood there would be setbacks on our road to research funding, and we tried to use the news about Geron to drive our efforts, not deter them. Meanwhile, I pushed ahead with "The Human Candidate" and tried to figure out where to include this unexpected event in the story outline. Between work and family and my commitment to our push for TJ's Law, writing time was precious and my life became an even more difficult balancing act. I quickly realized, however, that each step was necessary in order to convey the story accurately.

After putting the children to bed that evening, I took my computer to the front porch and wrote until after midnight. Somehow I was able to finish a fourth chapter, to Mac's pleasure. "This is EXACTLY the voice we are after!" He told me and asked that I keep him updated about any major developments with the clinical trial and with our campaign.

Indeed, things were moving quickly for our group. TJ was back in nursing school at the University of South Alabama and studying hard for winter exams. While Marc, Roman, and I were building a timeline for the campaign, we agreed that we didn't need to share details of the bill until after the Christmas holidays. In the meantime, Marc contacted a friend at the Alabama Department of Public Safety who ran numbers to determine the amount of money that would be generated from a surcharge applied to traffic violations. This was the revenue mechanism used in Roman's Law in California and had been a very effective and highly supported strategy to fund research there. With 35 percent of all spinal cord injuries caused by vehicular accidents—making them the leading cause of SCI—we agreed this should be the same funding strategy behind TJ's Law.

Using Roman's Law as a template for Marc's bill, this legislation would include a $1 fine for basic moving violations; a $5 fine for aggravated violations, such as reckless driving or following too closely; and a $10 fine for driving under the influence of alcohol. These fines would be tacked on to the existing state fines for these traffic violations. Based on the numbers given to Marc, we learned that TJ's Law could potentially raise up to $500,000 a year for research in Alabama. He was encouraged by these figures and felt certain his fellow legislators would see our initiative as an opportunity to increase state revenue and bring research awareness.

Marc planned to introduce his bill to key political figures in the weeks leading up to February 7, 2012, when the general legislative session reconvened in Montgomery. Until then, he would finalize the language and pre-file the bill soon after the first of the year. We spent time over the holidays doing as much research as possible, so that when it was time to announce the legislation, we would feel confident in our answers and be able to persuade constituents and legislators to support TJ's Law.

Also important at this time, Dr. Candace Floyd of UAB enthusiastically joined our team. After reading a draft of Marc's bill, she was quick to recommend we remove any language about human embryonic stem cell research, as it was an "understood" policy at UAB that this controversial research would not be publicly promoted. She had also been approached by other researchers in hopes their studies on traumatic brain injury could benefit from our funding, but we decided to focus solely on spinal cord injury research so the funding would not become diluted. Candace let our group know that, if given the opportunity, she would happily serve as the director of the TJ Atchison Spinal Cord Injury Research Program.

With much to discuss after Candace's feedback, Marc and I met the following day to finalize the language of the bill, along with deciding the best location to announce TJ's Law. We went back and forth about locations in both Birmingham and Mobile, as each had compelling value—Mobile and the USA campus there would surely be the better place to accommodate TJ's family and friends, while Marc reasoned that a press conference in Birmingham would be better attended. So we decided to hold a second conference at UAB campus later in February or in March. "After all, introducing TJ's bill is the simple part. It will take a monumental effort and multiple press conferences across our state to make this bill a reality," Marc explained.

I also called Roman on my way back to the office to talk about Candace's recommendation that we remove "human embryonic stem cell research" from the bill and replace it with "most efficacious method of treatment." Roman understood, and felt that we faced a much stronger chance of not gathering support for the bill if we did not modify the language. With this alternative verbiage inserted into the bill, researchers would still be allowed to conduct human embryonic stem cell research at UAB, but with the understanding that their research was using the "most efficacious method of treatment." We all understood that dreams must pass through the reality of action, and be ready to shift direction at any moment.

On January 30, 2012, before a crowd of fifty family members and friends, Senator Marc Keahey stood on the steps of USA's Moulton Tower and announced his plan to introduce the TJ Atchison Spinal Cord Injury Research Act in the Alabama state legislature. Although my children were in school and unable to attend the event, I was happy that my mother had been able to make it to our first press event. Mom sat in the front row with her arm around Anita and held TJ's little sister Alyssa in her lap. Mom's smile radiated from the crowd, and her pride brightened the gray skies above. After explaining the framework behind TJ's Law, the senator passed the microphone to TJ. With a smile across his face and a determined tone in his voice, he read from a crinkled piece of paper in his lap:

> Good afternoon! I am TJ Atchison, the world's first participant in our nation's first-ever federally approved clinical trial using human embryonic stem cell therapy and coauthor of "The Human Candidate." I am paralyzed from a car accident and fighting for a cure for paralysis.
>
> In firmly believing in the love, grace and sovereignty of God in creating and embracing human life, I also believe in the justification for sustaining a quality of life for myself, the 1.8 million Americans living with spinal cord injury paralysis, the 5.6 million Americans suffering from some form of paralysis, and for all people everywhere living paralyzed. It is my desire to convey a message of hope and peace and provide answers for why I decided to participate in the highly controversial clinical trial that began on October 8, 2010.
>
> So now I ask for your help in making the dreams of a paralysis cure a reality by supporting the TJ Atchison Spinal Cord Injury Research Act authored by our great Senator Marc Keahey!

> Our Law will impose a small $1 added surcharge on all moving traffic violations, $5 for aggravated moving violations, and $10 for DUI—no taxes, or state general fund withdrawals—to fund the research for a paralysis cure while creating jobs and giving hope to the paralyzed, all right here within our great home state of Alabama.
>
> Your support will strongly impact whether or not I spend the rest of my life confined to a wheelchair or achieve my dream of walking again. We must fund the research for spinal cord injury cure.
>
> I ask you: PLEASE STAND WITH ME, SO WE CAN ALL STAND WITH YOU!

And then, it was Roman's turn. "The very first mention of paralysis," he began, "was written inside the walls of an Egyptian tomb. It read, 'deny the paralyzed soldier water, for there is nothing that can be done.' For too long, that was the truth, but not now. Not anymore! There is MUCH that can be done, that WILL be done, and SHOULD be done." Quoting one of his boyhood heroes, Jackie Robinson, Roman reminded the crowd that, "A life is not worth living, EXCEPT for the impact it has on others."

In closing the press conference, Roman read from a letter written to him shortly after his football injury by the late Christopher Reeve, who turned despair into courage, and hope. "One day Roman and I shall stand up from our wheelchairs and walk away from them forever." Before the hushed crowd Roman finished: "Now that day did not come in time for our Superman, but with your help [defining the audience], the cure will happen."

As the afternoon came to an end and the crowd slowly disappeared into the pale winter light, I was so proud of Marc, our knight in shining armor, and of our brave TJ for speaking before a large crowd for the very first time. And I was grateful to the incredible Roman Reed for making the trip back to Alabama to share in this beautiful day, and for the opportunities before us to build both health and community, not only for ourselves, but for future generations.

16

TJ'S LAW BECOMES A REALITY

Montgomery and Birmingham, Alabama
February–March 2012

The week after our press conference in Mobile, I was thrilled to report back to the team that my phone had been ringing off the hook from supporters of TJ's Law. Many of the callers had requested a sample letter of support for the TJ Atchison Spinal Cord Injury Research Act and asked where it could be sent.

I drafted a sample letter of support, which included contact information for Senator Keahey. With the 2012 legislative session beginning the following day, the sooner those emails and ground letters went out the better, so I maximized our potential social media exposure by sharing the letter on Facebook, Twitter, and my blog.

A week later, we were amazed at the support shown for our initiative. Hundreds of letters poured into Senator Keahey's office, and hundreds more reached other legislators across the state.

Marc introduced the bill, SB338, into the Alabama senate on February 16, 2012. If enacted, the bill would create a spinal cord injury research program at the University of Alabama at Birmingham with an appointed director responsible for administering and awarding grants for spinal cord injury research within the program. In his first draft of SB338, Marc included that funding would come from imposing additional fees to certain traffic violations. However, because this research potentially affected so many more areas—medicine, education, the state economy—Marc had received bipartisan support to embed a $400,000 line item in the education trust fund budget for the TJ Atchison Spinal Cord Injury Research Program. This meant that the research would not only advance our knowledge of the spinal cord, but it would also support postdoctoral research and encourage the best and brightest young scientists in the field of spinal cord injury research to come to our state. It was a confirmation by both Democrats and Republicans of just how important this legislation was to Alabama.

So taking the advice of his colleagues, Marc introduced a new draft of SB338, and we were thrilled to hear that it was gaining support in the state legislature. In Alabama, as each legislative arm—senate and house of representatives—takes up a new piece of legislation, it goes to senate committee first, and if supported there, it will then be voted on by the entire senate floor a few weeks later. Then, the process repeats in the house of representatives—first in committee, then to a floor vote. Happily, and to our surprise and pleasure, our bill was assigned to the Alabama Senate Judiciary Committee, where Marc felt confident his strong relationships with committee members would work to our advantage of SB338 passing.

Sharing in our momentum and excitement, Dr. Candace Floyd invited me to tour her lab at UAB and hoped we could sit down and have a critical assessment of what she could do to help our efforts. She requested to meet with me privately, then coordinate a follow-up meeting with the entire group. I thought this approach was a nice gesture and a wonderful opportunity for me to learn more about existing spinal cord injury research at UAB.

After celebrating my oldest daughter's eleventh birthday with a house filled with preteen girls and boys from our town, I cleaned up the cake and decorations, waved good-bye to our guests, then packed the children for an overnight visit with my parents so I could meet with Candace at UAB the following day.

I made it to Birmingham late Saturday evening and met Candace for Sunday brunch at a nearby restaurant in Forest Park. We talked about her vision for expanding translational research (applying knowledge from basic science and translating it into meaningful health outcomes) at UAB. We then tossed around ideas for collaborating with successful programs across the United States. With only a few hours remaining in my trip, Candace drove us to the UAB campus and gave me a quick tour of the Spain Rehabilitation Center where she served as research director for the Department of Physical Medicine and Rehabilitation. I was introduced to many new medical terms and amazed to learn that UAB was home to the nation's oldest spinal cord injury "model system." Candace explained that in order to study a disease or injury in great depth, model systems were created so researchers could use the experience of the past (in that disease or injury) to build on in the future. This information would contribute to a body of knowledge in that model system, which in turn allows researchers to answer important questions about the disease or injury.

Established in 1972, UAB's spinal cord injury model system was one of fourteen such centers nationwide and was conceived and funded through a competitive federal grant program established by the National Institute on Disability and Rehabilitation Research. NIDRR awards SCI Model Systems Center grants in five-year cycles to institutions that are national leaders in medical research and patient care and strive to maintain and improve medical care for persons who incur spinal cord injuries.

UAB's SCI model system focused on rehabilitation research, not cure research. That meant that TJ's Law could be a game changer by expanding the focus of clinical research to include studies for both potential treatments and cures for spinal cord injury. If enacted by the state, this new program created and funded through the TJ Atchison Spinal Cord Injury Research Act would have immediate impact at UAB by accelerating research for paralysis cures.

Another incentive for distributing the appropriated funds from the TJ Atchison SCI Research Act to UAB was its ability to leverage resources through the established infrastructure. California's UC-Irvine, Stanford University, and UC-Davis were leading centers in the United States for research and discovery of novel treatments for SCI. Candace considered these centers as the premier locations for SCI treatments because they supported many jobs, obtained much federal funding, and had substantially accelerated the pace for clinical research. Candace had established relationships with her peers at these facilities in California and felt confident they would be willing to share their insights into the successes and failures of their programs.

We wrapped up the tour by discussing her need for an administrative assistant in her department. Candace asked if I was interested in such a position and encouraged me to consider joining her team at the Department of Physical Medicine and Rehabilitation. I was flattered and asked about the position's requirements. She laughed and said, "Based on my observations, Tory, you have exceeded all of them and would be considered a strong candidate for an AA in my department. There will be speaking engagements, event planning, and other responsibilities similar to what you're doing now, but most importantly, you will oversee the operation of TJ's new program and make certain we meet milestones for each year of funding from the state. You should update your resume and compile a portfolio of recommendation letters. There is a lengthy process we will have to go through with UAB's Human Resources Department, but when the position becomes available online, I'll invite you to submit an application for our review. How does that sound?"

My heart jumped because I had certainly not expected leaving Birmingham with a potential job offer. I had a lot to consider on my drive home to Millry. At the midway point in Tuscaloosa, I called my mom and described my day with Candace.

Mom was excited to hear how confident I felt that UAB would be the perfect location to house TJ's program. The idea of my relocating for a new job working with Candace, of course, was more complicated. Mom had questions as to what a job like this would entail. She would hate to lose us—a relocation would put us a three-hour drive away from her—but there was also so much more involved. I had to consider the cost of relocation, job stability, babysitting, and the challenge of shuttling kids to school and activities. How would that all work?

"Let's not worry about this now, Mom," I said. "All of this is in the future, maybe." And this was the truth. Right now I could not allow myself to become swept up by the distractions of the "what-ifs." I knew there were other pressing issues that had to be dealt with before even considering a position with Candace: I had to focus on our campaign for TJ's Law, and finish writing "The Human Candidate."

On February 29, SB338 was voted on and unanimously passed by the Senate Judiciary Committee. Once passed through the entire senate floor the following week, Representative Elaine Beech of Washington County would sponsor the bill in house committee where it, too, would be voted on and hopefully passed by the entire house floor. The bill would then be sent to Governor Bentley for signature. Marc and Elaine once again anticipated no opposition and hoped to pass the bill no later than May 1.

From March 6 through 8, I chaperoned a small group of teenagers who had been selected as Youth Tour representatives from Clarke-Washington Electric Membership Corporation (CWEMC) where I served as communication's director. Youth Tour was a highly regarded youth program in Clarke, Washington, Monroe, and Wilcox counties. Each year CWEMC sponsored several eleventh-grade students to attend the Montgomery Youth Tour. We joined other representatives from rural electric cooperatives throughout Alabama on this three-day trip to Montgomery, where we toured historic sites and met with leaders at the state capitol.

During our day trip to meet with legislators, I asked Marc if he could spend time with our group and explain the legislative process. Standing at the back of the conference room during Marc's presentation, I spotted Representative Mac McCutcheon and Representative Micky Hammon walk past our door, both key Republican lawmakers whose support I knew we needed for TJ's Law to pass in the house committee. Still to this day, I have no idea where my courage came from, but I slipped out the rear door, covered my Youth Tour badge with my hair, and purposely bumped into both representatives standing near the elevator.

"Hello, Representatives McCutcheon and Hammon. Please allow me to introduce myself to you."

Mac McCutcheon raised his hand to shake mine and asked, "How can I help you?"

I knew I didn't have but a few seconds to ask of his support for SB338, so I took a deep breath and poured my heart and soul into every word that left my mouth.

"Thank you, Sir. It is an honor to meet you. My name is Tory Minus [I kept my married name through months of separation and divorce, which was finalized two months later] and I would like to share with you my support of Senator Keahey's legislation SB338. With help from both you and Representative Hammon, it is our goal to get this important bill on the agenda and passed before the 2012 session ends."

Representative Hammon leaned forward and said, "I've heard about this bill. It's for spinal cord injury research, correct?"

"Yes, Sir. For over a year, I have devoted my time to help TJ Atchison bring awareness about spinal cord injury research to our state. In the last month, I have aligned with Senator Keahey and other supporters to get the TJ Atchison Spinal Cord Injury Research Act signed into law.

It's too important, and I will help in any way that I can along with great leaders like you and Representative McCutcheon who stand up for TJ and others who cannot yet stand!"

The elevator doors opened just as I finished my pitch. Representatives McCutcheon and Hammon both assured me they would support SB338 and help Senator Keahey get this legislation on the special agenda for next week's vote.

I was elated and could not wait to tell Marc this great news. There were other influential legislators I had hoped to bump into while in Montgomery, but for now, I had planted a seed with two that would carry heavy weight with their colleagues during the house committee vote. I slipped back inside the conference room and caught Marc staring in my direction with a curious grin across his face. He knew very well I had been up to something and hurried his talk with the Youth Tour kids so he could find out what I'd done.

Although he cautioned me for speaking with representatives while on the clock for Youth Tour, he was happy to hear I had seized the opportunity to lobby both McCutcheon and Hammon. That night, feeling flushed with energy, I coordinated a visit from my hotel room for our campaign team to meet the SCI researchers at the Spain Rehabilitation Center. Things indeed were moving swiftly. It had been only four months since Roman, TJ, Marc, and I had met and created a plan for TJ's Law. As it appeared we were nearing our goal, I felt it was time to jump-start the next piece of action, securing a SCI program at UAB. I was delighted Roman would catch a red-eye from California to join us in Birmingham.

Just before lunch, Dr. Candace Floyd introduced some notable UAB administrators and staff: Dr. Richard Marchase, professor and vice president of Research and Economic Development, and Dr. Robert Kimberly, professor and senior associate dean for research, as well as many key members of the Department of Physical Medicine and Rehabilitation. Everyone was tremendously excited by what the pending legislative bill would mean to UAB's research team. As Dr. Marchase said, "This legislation is very important for all Alabamians living with spinal cord injury, and we will be great stewards of the funds generated from it." Not only was our meeting a great opportunity to bring together fellow supporters of spinal cord injury research, it was the perfect forum for learning more about the incredible work being done at UAB and for exchanging innovative ideas of how to make this important research a priority in our state. It was a day filled with motivation and new friendships, all around a common goal to get the paralyzed out of their chairs and back on their feet.

The following day, back from Birmingham, I emailed our literary agent Mac Mackie and asked for an update with our book proposal for "The Human Candidate," then on submission to various editors. Although the material was still under consideration by seven houses, we were definitely seeing a frustrating trend: the bigger houses thought our book was too religious to take on for their general trade lists, and the religious publishers believed that the topic of stem cell research was too controversial for their lists. Each type of publisher was recommending the other. We were falling somehow into the proverbial no-man's land.

TJ's and my frustration grew; however, we understood that it was a very difficult line to straddle. Could we have eliminated the faith-based aspect of the story in order to appeal to those larger houses? Not really. TJ's faith gave credence to the story's impact and purpose. And honestly, the energetic advocacy for research and flair for promotion one associated with Roman Reed, Michael J. Fox, and Christopher Reeve was just not going to be TJ's thing. He was uninterested in participating in social media or in the idea of crisscrossing the country for book promotion, interviews, speaking engagements, and large public events. As for the religious publishers, we pushed the material for another month, but, inevitably, they felt the topic would turn off too many of their readers. Conservative America was still unready to listen to our truth.

Sadly, I realized that time is measured by seasons only, and our season for this book had not yet arrived. With disappointment come compensations, and deep cleansing breaths. It became obvious to me that we should focus on TJ's Law, and if the book were meant to be published, the right editor and publishing house would find us at the right time. TJ and I were sorry to see our relationship with Mac come to an end.

There was little time to grieve the breakup with Mac or hold on to our book project as news from Senator Keahey came on May 16 that funding for the TJ Atchison Spinal Cord Injury Research Program had been approved by the Alabama state legislature and was expected to be signed by Governor Bentley very soon. With pride and elation, I announced on my blog that this initiative would provide approximately $400,000 annually in research funding to the University of Alabama Birmingham School of Medicine.

The money would be administered by Dr. Candace Floyd, interim director of clinical research for the Department of Physical Medicine and Rehabilitation. "This is an important initiative that will go a long way toward finding a cure and alleviating the side effects that spinal cord injury patients experience," she said for our post on my blog.

Marc said in his official press release, "I am honored to bring the TJ Atchison Spinal Cord Injury Research Program to the forefront of Alabama's innovative medical research efforts." He added, "This is cutting edge research, and I feel Alabama will benefit from having it on hand."

For Marc, TJ, Roman, and me, having the support of the Alabama legislature and gaining the support of constituents across the state meant we would remain energized and focused on strengthening research in Alabama and across the world. Giving all the glory to God: WE DID IT!

17

MOVING MOUNTAINS

Millry and Birmingham, Alabama
June–November 2012

After TJ's Law passed into law in May, our same group—TJ, Marc, Roman, and I—teleconferenced each Sunday to monitor the new program's progress at UAB. Candace was busy organizing an internal advisory board consisting of deans, administrators, and faculty from the academic institution. This board helped create, among other tasks, a mission statement and established a timetable for the days and weeks leading up to October 1, when the TJ Atchison Spinal Cord Injury Program would officially launch.

With the establishment of our spinal cord research program, that summer saw an outpouring of support and interest from thousands across the state who suffered from spinal cord injuries. And with this great momentum came many opportunities—opportunities which left Candace in dire need of a management team to assist her in these new endeavors.

So in late July, Candace officially invited me to submit my resume and letters of recommendation for the position of educational liaison and program administrator for TJ's program. In her email, she provided information regarding the job's requirements and salary range, along with a health benefits package.

Unfortunately, the position and salary range had to be signed off by UAB's Human Resources Department, which had determined that an annual salary above $60,000—which I would need because of the cost of living in Birmingham, so much higher than Millry—would require a job candidate to hold a doctorate degree. And, because I did not have this type degree, I did not believe I could uproot my children and resign from my current job that provided financial stability to take a position that could not sustain my family in Birmingham.

Candace was frustrated but still encouraged me to apply and offered an option of working remote from Millry until I could afford to make a permanent move. I was disappointed too, as I had already decided that I wanted to work with Candace to help her build this special program. After all, I had already sacrificed so much to help TJ and Roman; my heart was telling me to go for it, but my head was telling me to think smart and not overextend myself financially. My parents and I prayed for direction and assurance that a move to Birmingham was the right decision for my family to make.

We were still waiting for the funding for the position with Candace at UAB to come through, and I was extremely nervous about making a final decision to move, so I turned to Roman for advice. He had known Candace for over a decade and was optimistic that it was the right professional move for me and that everything would work out if I decided to take the plunge and go for it. A few days later, Roman called and told me that if I accepted the position with Candace and relocated to Birmingham, he and his friends in California would help with my rent until I secured extra income. I reached out to a friend who in turn was able to direct me to a freelance writing job that added an extra thousand dollars to my monthly income. Even though the idea of working two jobs seemed torturous, I knew that if I stayed healthy and mentally strong, I could handle the tight deadlines and extra work in addition to my responsibilities at UAB.

Because I had nearly two weeks of vacation days remaining with my current employer, I decided to take several days off from work to find a rental property we could move into in time for my children to begin school August 20. The kids and I made a weekend visit to Birmingham and became quite fond of the Liberty Park subdivision, school campus, and the beautiful nature trails that were saturated with white-tailed deer and other wildlife.

I emailed Candace the following Monday and told her about our weekend visit. She was thrilled that the children enjoyed the city and that we had found an area where we wanted to live. That same day, she put me in contact with her friend Anne, a Birmingham realtor, who spent the next week helping me find several rental properties in Liberty Park that worked within my budget.

On August 1, Anne was successful in negotiating a great deal for a lease-to-own home in Liberty Park. That evening, the kids and I invited my parents and siblings over for a discussion of our move. It was definitely bittersweet leaving those we loved and all that was familiar to us in Washington County, especially when most of our family was there, along with a job I adored, my beautiful home on my parent's property, and a church group and school we loved.

But we knew God had a bigger plan for us; everything was falling into place, so this must be His plan. So after countless back porch conversations with my mom and sister, I felt a tremendous sense of peace about this huge change we were about to make. The children were terribly excited to meet new friends and have access to a movie theater, restaurants, a shopping mall, parks, and a community swimming pool, all within walking distance from our neighborhood. Their enthusiasm was confirmation from above that this was the right decision for my family.

On August 13, Catie and I stuffed our last box into the U-Haul and walked from room to room, reminiscing about our years in Millry. There had been so much activity in our lives during those weeks leading up to our move that everything did not really sink in until that final evening. We said our good-byes to family and friends through a fine rain of tears the following morning, but there was also excitement in our hearts as we drove away and thought of making a fresh start in Birmingham. We were ready for the adventure and eager to make a difference in the lives of others, and for ourselves.

A week after settling into our new home, the kids shot out the door for their first day of school with absolutely zero trouble. Little Courtney made new friends easily, and Carlie and Conner skipped away from me as if starting a new school was no biggie. Catie was a little nervous, but eager to get the day going at Liberty Park Middle School. I watched her walk away from me, her pink top sparkling in the bright morning light and complementing her summer tan and long, dark hair. How quickly my children were growing up, as I was too.

My parents surprised the children and me that afternoon by making the trip to Birmingham for an overnight visit. We were super excited to show them around the area. Mom and Dad expressed how proud they were of us all for being so brave in our new surroundings. They, too, fell quickly in love with the neighborhood and their short planned visit turned into a week's stay. Extending their time with us in fact allowed them to accompany Catie and me to Montgomery for the ceremonial bill signing of TJ's Law.

On August 31, 2012, Representative Elaine Beech, friends, family, and supporters of TJ, along with Dr. Candace Floyd and other UAB staff joined Governor Bentley and the legislation's author, Senator Marc Keahey, for a ceremonial bill signing at the capitol. My parents, Catie, and I were so tremendously pleased to share this special day with TJ and his family.

We knew that Governor Bentley was extremely busy and had many things on his agenda, such as visiting the families of south Alabama who had been affected by tropical storm Isaac earlier in the week. We expected the ceremony would be quick; however, when the governor came to meet us in the beautiful old office chamber room of the capitol, he took great time to speak with TJ and me about our goals for this program, and then asked others in our group if they had any questions for him.

My daughter Catie and TJ's sister Alyssa also had alone time with the governor. He held the hands of our little ones and encouraged them to be great students and friends, and to work hard in their schools and communities. When there were no more picture requests or questions left to ask, the governor seated himself at a desk in the center of the room and we gathered around him for the bill-signing ceremony. TJ turned and looked at me over his right shoulder. His smile brought tears to my eyes because we knew that, together, we had accomplished something truly amazing.

The next month flew by quickly, as I was busy with freelance writing and planning several fundraisers for TJ in Birmingham. We also celebrated my thirty-fifth birthday. Then came the hoped-for phone call from Candace inviting me to interview for the educational liaison position at TJ's program. The funding had finally been approved, and the position looked favorably mine, or so we all hoped. During the interview, I presented my progress with a charitable golf tournament that I was organizing for the following April, along with other ideas for raising funds and awareness for TJ's program. I also shared several letters of recommendations from influential personal supporters including Senator Keahey, Roman Reed, Dr. Hans Keirstead, and my previous employer at CWEMC.

Candace and the interview panel were impressed with my presentation, and on the spot offered me the position of educational liaison for TJ's program. As my vehicle had just been threatened for repossession, and with the recent notification that our family health insurance would expire at the end of the month, it was a tremendous relief to hear their offer. There was no plan B in place and very little in savings to keep my family in Birmingham beyond another week or two. This was a life-changing moment, and I vowed to give this new opportunity everything I had.

My first day of work at UAB was October 9, 2012. When I had met with Candace for the first time back in February, a position with her had been thousands of miles away in my mind. I had climbed many mountains to find myself where I was today, and I found myself once again giving thanks to God for the glorious team He had sent my way—from the awesome Senator Marc Keahey, whom my father mentored during his launch into politics, to TJ, an inspiration and friend of my family, and Candace, whom Roman was honored to have funded a decade before and was scientifically impressed by for years. I had traveled light-years. It still amazed me how I had journeyed away from the risk-averse housewife to become someone who believed with all her heart that life's fullness lies in the leaps we take. And so I marveled.

From my family's move to the big city three hours away from the safety and predictability of our homestead and support group to a hoped-for job with Candace, all without a written offer of employment in place. I was taking risks that were unimaginable before this journey began two years before. Thankfully I also had Roman's generous promise that he would help me every step of the way as my safe place to land. I only hoped I could contribute positively to this amazing program.

When I walked the halls of UAB during those first days, taking time to speak with the patients at the Spain Rehabilitation Center, I felt honored to be a part of something so great and glorious. Now, both as a single mother and as an emerging advocate for stem cell research, I made a promise to myself and family to never fail at helping others.

On November 13, over a hundred people gathered at UAB's North Pavilion Atrium for the open house and ribbon cutting ceremony for the TJ Atchison Spinal Cord Injury Research Program.

The event began with a warm welcome and introductions by Dr. Amie McLain, professor and chair of the Department of Physical Medicine and Rehabilitation. Prerecorded greetings were shown from Dr. Marchase, UAB's interim president, and from Dr. Kimberly. Candace provided a PowerPoint, which explained the vision, mission, and goals for TJ's program, followed by Roman, who had returned to us once again and whose powerful message of advocacy and perseverance demonstrated his passion and motivation for raising awareness and funding for spinal cord injury research.

TJ, visibly overwhelmed with gratitude for the support and guidance he had received over the last two years and the efforts by so many to bring us to this day, took the microphone and thanked the crowd for attending this special event. Closing remarks were given by Marc Keahey, who touched my heart by recognizing me as "the force behind it all."

Just an hour prior to this wonderful celebration, TJ had called to order the first steering committee meeting of his newly established foundation. Founding members of this nonprofit organization included TJ, Roman, Marc's wife Lara Keahey (my good friend from back home), Bonnie Blackwell (who had become paralyzed after a car accident in 2005), and me. Indeed we had many goals for the TJ Atchison Foundation, including an expansive vision for spinal cord injury research that incorporated grant opportunities for new researchers, as well as other initiatives to support our cause.

The week following the ribbon cutting ceremony and foundation launch, I was moving at lightning speed to meet with various department heads before the start of winter break crept in. After coordinating several meetings with top administrators across the School of Medicine, I noticed that many of the UAB researchers were interested in learning how Roman and I had teamed up together and helped Senator Keahey pass TJ's Law in the Alabama legislature. They asked if there was anything I could do to help raise awareness and funding for their particular research areas, which energized an idea that had been brewing inside my head for several weeks.

Indeed, I thought they were right. What if there was a program in place across our state to help researchers advance their novel ideas, specifically those related to stem cell technology? So, the week before Thanksgiving holiday I made two phone calls to my dearest friends and allies. Marc and Roman both knew that when I gave them a call without emailing or texting first, something was in the works. For thirty minutes, I explained my plan to fund research that would target and hopefully eliminate every disease known to man.

To many this goal would seem unreachable, but not to Marc, Roman, and me. With their support and involvement in this initiative, I knew there were no limits to what we could accomplish. We were on the right track and *aimed for cures*!

18

THE PERFECT MATCH

Birmingham, Alabama
November 2012

Just before Thanksgiving, my daughter Catie caught a television commercial for Match.com, a popular online dating service connecting men and women. Because many of these relationships resulted in engagement and marriage, Catie teasingly encouraged me to create a profile and join. I was reluctant for many reasons, but especially because we had been through so much in less than one year that I felt our family dynamics were finally somewhat grounded again.

I had not dated much in the two years since my marriage ended in 2011. But after much consideration and becoming increasingly tired of being teased by friends as a hermit crab, I took Catie's advice and registered. My first week on Match.com seemed like a total waste of time, as I was receiving winks and inbox messages from all of the wrong types of men. I seriously doubted my "soulmate" could be just a few clicks away and contemplated removing my profile from the site.

However, one week later, while scouting sponsors for TJ's golf tournament, I heard a ding on my phone and had time between appointments to check out the notification. It was a response to a profile picture I had liked on Match.com for a ronwilliams77. Ron's photo appealed to me because of his warm smile and the tight bear hug he was giving a child, who I'd learn later was his oldest son. The photo somehow gave me the urge to connect. Ron's profile was by far the most interesting that I had stumbled across—he enjoyed adventure, travel, philanthropy, and most importantly, FAMILY. He was also a risk-taker and an entrepreneur who shared my interest in the medical field.

After two email exchanges and one fifteen-minute phone conversation, we decided to meet. So on November 29, I waited nervously for him to pick me up at the Spain Rehabilitation Center. I was early and decided to walk around the corner of Eighteenth Street and Sixth Avenue South to pass time until he arrived. I checked my reflection in the windows and adjusted my hair and outfit. Everything seemed in place, but I was as nervous as a schoolgirl.

There were no parking spots in front of the Spain Rehab building, so Ron improvised by parking in a loading zone on Nineteenth Street. He called my cell and offered to walk across the street to find me, but based on the description he gave of his truck, I spotted him and was already walking in his direction. Our eyes caught one another and he smiled, immediately erasing my fears. He was sweet to apologize for not being able to open the door for me, but with lunch hour traffic at its peak, cars raced past us, so I jumped into the passenger seat and we sped away.

During our drive to lunch, Ron and I had a good initial connection, and the conversation was fun and light. I had heard great things about the restaurant he'd selected for our first meeting. We made our way inside Bottega and found a quiet spot in the back corner. There was a definite physical chemistry between us, and I was hoping he was as charming, witty, and intellectual as his profile insinuated. After an hour lunch, followed by another hour as we lingered over coffee, Ron and I agreed that we shared many common interests—stem cell research and helping others, and for both of us, our children were the top priorities in our lives.

The youngest of four children, Ron was raised in the small Louisiana town of Clinton, some thirty miles north of Baton Rouge, where he spent the majority of his teenage years helping in the family-owned restaurant called the Front Porch. I was fascinated to learn that his father had invented a popular injectable marinade called The Cajun Injector. Ron smiled as he reminisced about his childhood and explained that he had learned a lot from his parents about a hard-work ethic and accountability. His father impressed this lesson most: that if you're up past 10 p.m., then you're probably doing something you shouldn't be doing. And from his mother, Ron learned the importance of believing that he could do anything if he set his mind to it.

After two years at Louisiana State University, a very restless Ron dropped out of college, to his parent's disappointment, and briefly ran his own restaurant, naming it Ron's Corner Cafe, before moving on to Dallas, Texas, where he worked for a prominent family who owned over ninety restaurants nationwide. Ron worked as a manager, trainer, and even created recipes for their popular menu. He worked longer hours than anyone and restructured the restaurant's service so that patrons received quicker response and at a better price. Promotion after promotion, Ron was encouraged by his supervisor to think bigger and broader than the restaurant industry, so he reached out to an old friend who had advanced to senior management in sales. A few phone calls later, Ron was on a plane heading to New Jersey to interview with a vice president of Stryker, the medical equipment supplier, for a sales representative position. The executive was impressed with Ron's outgoing personality and tenacious spirit, in spite of Ron's lack of a college degree. It was the one chance the ambitious young man needed.

Fast-forward five years later: with a young family in tow, he accepted a position to transfer to Birmingham so he could move his wife closer to her parents before the birth of their first child. As the years passed quickly, Ron became immersed in the competitive spirit of medical sales, working eighty-hour weeks, which helped him break several sales records and rise to the top at remarkable speed. Through his years with Stryker, Ron watched medicine change for the better and health care for the worse. He believed the future of the economics around our nation's health care crisis lay in the new stem cell therapies. We talked and talked, clearly finding we had much in common. Leaving the restaurant and walking to his truck, I noticed his license plate read "ICABLZ," and asked him what that meant.

He smiled sweetly and said "I is me, and CABLZ is my company." It turned out that Ron had invented an eyewear retainer system in 2008 called CABLZ that attaches on both ends of a pair of glasses, keeping them safe and off the neck. He said it had taken many months of hard work to launch this unique product, but in just eighteen months, his

CABLZ was global. He was most proud that, in 2009, this invention was recognized by the International Convention of Allied Sportfishing Trades (ICAST) as a new product showcase winner.

This was a lot to take in for our first meeting, but stepping down from his truck I knew that I only wanted to know more. I certainly felt there was potential for something great between us and hoped he felt the same. With his passenger window rolled down, he asked for my availability of getting together again the next week for dinner and a movie. I was thrilled that he wanted to see me again so soon. It was exciting that we both wanted to see where this new friendship could go.

Sure enough, a romance followed, unexpectedly but with a wonderful and spontaneous joy. I was thirteen years younger than Ron, who was also divorced and had concerns about pursuing a relationship with someone so many years younger. Both of our marriages had ended badly, in fact, and I was wary initially too. But having just turned the page to a new chapter in his life after going through his traumatic divorce—one that stretched over three years before being finalized—Ron had witnessed approximately twenty other divorces of close friends living within blocks of his home. He explained this as the "forty- to fifty-year-old midlife-crisis epidemic that seemed to be as contagious as the common cold." And so foreign to my personal experience with divorce, Ron explained that the majority of these marriages ended because the woman left at a whim. "The reasons seemed to vary," he said, "but they were all superficial reasons that left the women with much fatter bank accounts than their ex-husbands."

I was happy to learn that Ron wanted a companion with depth, character, and an altruistic spirit. My heart filled with happiness when he explained that he found me refreshing and healing to his bruised heart. I, too, understood exactly what he meant and shared the same sentiment about him. Just after ringing in New Year's together, Ron and I believed we had found in each other a deeper understanding of how kindred spirits were truly able to connect through the most unlikely and adverse situations. After the strain and distance of our previous marriages, we basked in being loved so well. Ron drew me out again into the sunlight; our ease and passion for one another was a wonderful surprise. I embraced this new feeling of connectedness, like a warm wind blowing sweetly across a country field.

Spring 2013 moved in and brought great activity and pleasure to my life—a wonderful job, a new circle of friends, and a community in which Ron and our children flourished. TJ's program at UAB was moving seamlessly ahead—while that fledgling idea of mine, aided by Marc and Roman, was gaining support with researchers and administrators at the academic institute and across the state. My passion for helping others was about to take a broad turn.

19

AIM-4-CURES

Birmingham, Alabama
December 2012–April 2013

My office at the Spain Rehabilitation Center was directly across from a building that meant so much to my family and me. Children's of Alabama was the hospital where my sister Tera's life was saved so many years ago. I thanked God each day that she had won her battle with cancer and had been in remission since 1990.

Now, living as I was with polycystic kidney disease (PKD) and deeply involved with my work in the area of stem cell research and spinal cord injury, it was clear that scientists from across the state were not being encouraged to include progressive stem cell approaches—such as hESC, for example—in their studies. After meeting with dozens of patient advocates, political leaders, and researchers supporting regenerative medicine, I realized more could be done to help move science forward and put Alabama on the map as a leader in the field.

Because I was born into a family of community-doers and advocates for progress and change, it was sewn into my DNA to make a difference in areas needing a voice and support. And so in December 2012, I announced my plan to launch a new campaign called AIM-4-Cure, with the help and support of Roman and Marc and with, again, the encouragement of family and friends. The Alabama Institute of Medicine (AIM) was conceived as a new funding mechanism for advancing regenerative medicine in our state, not just for spinal cord injuries, but also for every disease and disability known to man.

I was certain that if successful, AIM would help fund the best science, create jobs, and bring enormous revenues to Alabama and its top research centers. With direct, leveraged, donated and matching grant funds drawing millions of dollars of research monies into the state, AIM would help UAB, in particular, be recognized as a national leader in medical research and cures.

But with this great opportunity came challenge, as I had to be careful not to jeopardize my job with Candace. Once again, I turned to Roman for ideas about bridging together AIM and my work at UAB. We developed two structures of AIM: First, we could mimic California's Prop 71, the 2004 bond initiative that supported a $3 billion research program named the California Institute of Regenerative Medicine. Through CIRM, hundreds of spin-off companies formed, thousands of jobs were created, and the California economy soared. Or we could establish AIM as a nonprofit organization that would raise funds and awareness for stem cell research at the university as well as at all accredited academic institutions and biotech companies across Alabama. Established as either a state program or a nonprofit organization, AIM funding would be disbursed to researchers through a competitive grant process: applicants would submit their proposals to AIM's scientific grant review committee for consideration, and this committee would then make funding recommendations to AIM's board of directors based on each proposal's scientific merit and requested budget. Priority would be given to human stem cell research and to other studies with clear potential relevance to human health, including animal models of human disease, regeneration, repair, and aging. The top scored research proposals would then be funded through AIM.

With UAB being the largest research institution in the state, I knew my campaign for AIM should begin there in order to gain administrative support and to eliminate any conflict of interest issues that could arise because of my involvement. So on January 7, I completed my first draft of a proposal to create AIM, and although this was not a requirement of my position at UAB, I submitted it to Candace for review. She was impressed by the material and recommended we develop the strategic plan a bit further before sharing it with our department chair and university administration.

After revising the proposal, I presented the new draft to Candace, which she forwarded along to our department chair, Dr. Amie McLain. We were thrilled when a few days later Dr. McLain met with us and gave her support and blessing to advancing our efforts for AIM. Dr. McLain moved quickly to contact her supervisors and to coordinate a meeting with key members of the university's administration, including Dr. Richard Marchase, Interim UAB president, and Dr. Ray Watts, dean of UAB's School of Medicine.

A week later, I accompanied Candace and Dr. McLain to a meeting at UAB Administration Building. We were escorted inside the main conference room, where Dr. McLain made the introductions to Dr. Watts and Dr. Marchase. Dr. McLain reminded both gentlemen that I had led the team which successfully established TJ's Law, and now we hoped to gain support for another initiative in our state to create the Alabama Institute of Medicine (AIM).

In a confident but respectful tone, I followed Dr. McLain's introduction and described what we hoped to do. I explained that since my recruitment to UAB, I had witnessed the talent and capabilities of the university staff, and believed AIM could provide additional resources and funding that were needed to achieve cures. This new program would accelerate the work being done in the laboratories and expedite these studies toward human clinical trials.

The administrators flipped through the proposal and jotted down notes as I talked. I could tell from the wide-eyed looks and nods exchanged across the conference table that both were intrigued with the material and information provided. It was an incredible feeling to think that AIM could gain their support and our new initiative could be pushed through with UAB behind us all the way.

Our meeting concluded with Dr. Watts requesting copies of detailed analytical reports on the economic impact and cash flow prepared for other states—California, Connecticut, Maryland, and others—with similar programs, specifically those that examined the financial impact of funding medical research as bond initiatives. He felt we had a good chance of gaining legislative support to make AIM a state program like CIRM.

The following day, Roman, Marc, Candace, and I teleconferenced with Don Reed and James Harrison, who had helped draft the legislative bill for Proposition 71. James answered our questions regarding the bond initiative used to generate funding for CIRM's $3 billion program.

He provided figures that could be adapted to show the positive impact for economic development and also explained how these hard, impressive numbers could possibly overshadow the potential sensitivities that the subject of stem cell research might arouse in our state.

On January 31, Roman flew to Alabama for important meetings with UAB researchers, community outreach coordinators, and disability rights groups. We were privileged to meet with Dr. Tim Wick and Dr. Joanne Murphy-Ullrich of the Biomatrix Engineering Regenerative Medicine (BERM) Center at UAB. The BERM Center's core mission focused on developing cell-based treatments and tissue replacement products and technologies. Also joining our meeting was Samantha Giordano, a UAB graduate student who volunteered to help build community support for our AIM campaign; and Victoria Allen, of the UAB Development Office.

We felt confident that information shared during this meeting would serve as a resource for Senator Keahey, who planned to file the bill to make AIM a state-funded program the following week. All he needed to move forward was UAB's official endorsement, along with that of the Governmental Affairs Office plus some additional information from California and Connecticut demonstrating the economic impact from their state-supported research programs. Marc believed he could persuade legislators to support AIM, but only if he could prove this research would boost the state's economy.

Our busy week of productive meetings had finally come to an end. I felt we were making great progress and was looking forward to a nice evening with my children and Ron's, along with several friends we'd invited over for a pre-launch celebration of AIM. The group included our close friends Sean and Dawn Hentz, Dr. Wick and his wife, and Dr. Murphy-Ullrich and her husband, along with AIM volunteer Samantha Giordano and her boyfriend.

We enjoyed a great meal, accompanied by several bottles of sparkling Pinot Grigio and deep Merlots, and finished with a delicious raspberry cream cheesecake and coffee. Ron toasted to our health, our children, our happiness, and to our dreams of living in a world free of disease and injury. We shut the feast down just before ten o'clock and said our good-byes with warm hugs and well wishes for the future of AIM. None of us, however, could have forecast the crosscurrents of events that would occur the following month.

On February 4, I coordinated a teleconference for Roman, Marc, James Harrison, Bob Klein, who was the spearhead of Prop 71 and founder of CIRM, and Senator Chris Murphy, who had sponsored similar legislation in Connecticut in 2006 supporting stem cell research. Our group discussed many topics, but key to the conversation, Senator Keahey wanted to learn more about the economic benefit Connecticut experienced from its stem cell research program.

Senator Murphy explained that the potential of stem cell research was incredible, and the potential benefits for Alabama specifically were significant. He said, "With no programs like this in place in the southeast, you will attract industry from neighboring states. From our experience, private investors and NIH are drawn to our stem cell research as well. Not a single person in Connecticut speaks out in opposition to our program. Our legislators have cut other sectors, but not this one because of the huge economic benefits our state receives each year from it. You can't get near this program when discussing budget cuts because of the amount of money it pours into our state. This kind of leveraging will be extremely important to you in Alabama. Stem cell research has definitely come into its own over the years in Connecticut and around the globe. Early on [during years one and two] it was just our private and state money supporting it, but since then, our program has grown thanks to both state and federal funding. In the last year, we attracted a major laboratory company called Jackson Labs to the state. They built a new facility that created hundreds if not thousands of jobs in Connecticut. This facility is right next to our stem cell lab and both are next to the University of Connecticut campus in Storrs. This company came to Connecticut for a number of reasons, but they will tell you that in most part they selected our state because of our stem cell labs and the research being done here. So, it's not only direct NIH dollars we are attracting, but also big bioscience companies, too, because they see our research and potential. You have the same potential in Alabama. There's plenty of funding and research interest to go around, including international support and investment opportunities."

Connecticut's Senator Murphy and California's Bob Klein assured Marc that he had their support and guidance, which would be crucial for moving AIM forward in the 2013 legislative session. We ended the teleconference by agreeing that Marc had the resources in place to file his bill in support of AIM. He voiced what a shame it would be if people in Alabama had to wait ten to fifteen years for stem cell treatments and care. "Through AIM," Marc said in concluding the call, "I believe there is hope our citizens will have early access to breakthroughs and therapies. Thank you all for your time today. I'll keep you updated on our progress."

As we moved into the second week of February, I grew concerned over Marc's hesitation to file his bill for AIM. Our local television stations and newspapers were slammed with what was forthcoming for the 2013 session, and there was no mention at all that a new stem cell research program was being sponsored. Information from a direct source at UAB indicated that a phone conversation between newly appointed UAB president Dr. Ray Watts (former dean of UAB School of Medicine) and Senator Keahey had occurred on February 13, and that the response Marc received from President Watts was positive, enthusiastic, and supportive of our proposal. It was our understanding that President Watts was going to take the idea to Chancellor Robert Witt of the University of Alabama system for his review and recommendation to move the legislation forward. But we also learned that a governmental relations official of the university had claimed that our AIM initiative would negatively affect the state's budget, which was totally untrue. In fact, the projections for AIM indicated significant increases in state revenue and research support for both UAB and research institutions across the state.

After a phone call with President Watts, Candace recommended that I email our supervisor, Dr. Amie McLain, with an update, which I gladly did.

In response, Dr. McLain reported that her contact at UAB indicated the university would not push for AIM as we had hoped, a major setback to be sure. We knew that without the university coming on board, the legislature would not either. However, Roman and I were prepared to go with plan B, just in case—we would launch AIM as a 501(c)(3) nonprofit organization and fund the grant program through public and private support.

AIM's planning committee (Roman, Samantha Giordano, Dr. Wick, and Dr. Murphy-Ullrich) in fact had requested information from UAB regarding the university's position with this research proposal. Because there were many potential donors and investors reaching out to request meetings with our AIM team, we were on a time crunch to determine whether AIM should move forward through state legislation or as a privately supported organization.

On March 5, I emailed President Watts with our options and asked for a few minutes to discuss our situation over the phone. During a quick lunch with Ron at his home in Vestavia Hills, President Watts called and expressed his appreciation to our group for developing such a strong concept for this new research program. Unfortunately, he reported that UAB and UA would like to focus for now on their internal fundraising campaign for the next four years and then work together to pass something state-funded for research after their efforts ended in 2017.

I respected his position, but explained that in that case, we did not want to wait four years, and we would proceed with AIM as a privately supported institute similar to St. Jude Children's Research Hospital.

Our planning committee believed stem cell research would advance the entire field of medicine, and we didn't want to wait and have our top researchers recruited away. We knew there was a significant economic benefit to keeping Alabama's best and brightest researchers and medical experts in-state rather than watching them leave along with the highly prized dollars they took with them. The most important point that I stressed to President Watts was that it was our goal to help Alabama citizens have the best available medical care nationwide.

President Watts commended my spirit and wished me great success with AIM. Throughout the remainder of March and into early April, I finalized plans for TJ's golf tournament to benefit his research program at UAB. I also took a few days away from the office to secure our final sponsors and collect goody bag items for the event. As chairperson of the tournament committee, it was my responsibility to make certain everything ran smoothly and that we reached our fundraising goal of $20,000. With two weeks remaining before the tournament, we still lacked a top tier sponsorship commitment, which we'd be offering for $15,000.

I was very concerned because without such a sponsorship, we would barely break even and have less than $5,000 to donate back into TJ's program. Knowing how much TJ and this program meant to me, Ron spent several days making calls to friends and was able to secure the $15,000 sponsorship for the tournament. He also pledged his company, CABLZ, as the golf cart sponsor and donated a pair of adjustable CABLZ to each golfer registered in the tournament. TJ and I were appreciative of Ron's generosity along with that of all the other sponsors who supported this inaugural fundraising event.

But back at the office, my relationship with Candace had begun to feel strained. There were several reasons for this. She had asked that I volunteer for another group, the Mike Jezdimir Foundation, which consisted of four patient advocates—Mike himself serving as chairman of the foundation—who had recently partnered to raise money for a rare spinal cord disease called transverse myelitis. Candace also requested that I assist them in the incorporation process of Mike's nonprofit organization, which was at the earliest stage of development.

I wanted to help Mike with his foundation, but to do so required additional hours of personal time and expenses for gas and babysitters that I just didn't have. I expressed my concerns to Candace about this and other unrelated job responsibilities that were becoming problematic, but I found no relief. In fact, the situation only worsened. Several employees in neighboring departments had either resigned, retired, or been reassigned. Instead of filling those positions with new employees, Candace asked that I step in, but without offering to modify my pay or my schedule. The extra physical, financial, and emotional burden, particularly at the expense of family time, was starting to wear me down.

As I was trying to juggle my full-time educational liaison position with Candace, the two foundations I was volunteering for—TJ's and Mike's—not to mention the complicated tasks involving the launch of AIM, this book I was writing about the quest to raise support and awareness for stem cell research, and now being asked to pick up the workload of former colleagues, I knew my life was not sustainable. Candace and I needed to talk. I was exhausted and could not do any more. I remained calm and spent several hours over the weekend to reflect and discuss my options with Ron, Roman, and of course my mother.

After careful consideration, I ultimately determined that AIM held priority over everything work-related, and I would turn in my notice of resignation to Candace the following Monday for my position at UAB.

It was a very, very difficult decision because I loved helping others and had found such purpose in my job at the Spain Rehabilitation Center. But I also knew I had to concentrate my efforts and do my most important job very well—making AIM work—or juggle them all and please no one, most of all myself. So on April 8, I approached Candace in a respectful and private manner in our office suite and explained my thinking. I asked her to please support my decision and know that I was resigning out of the highest consideration to TJ, his program at UAB, and the Department of Physical Medicine and Rehabilitation.

I wanted everything to be in proper order for my replacement, so I spent the next few days organizing files and making certain TJ's program material was efficiently documented and in an easy-to-find location. Most importantly, with the golf benefit only a week away, I wanted to reassure TJ and Anita that I was working hard to finalize the event plans. Each day leading up to the tournament, I averaged sixteen- to eighteen-hour workdays, busy wrapping up every loose end that remained with player registrations, sponsorships, budget, volunteers, giveaways, and day-of-event logistics. There was very little time for AIM planning, but I knew that soon I would be able to devote every waking minute to building this new and glorious organization to its greatest potential.

With Candace away at a workshop in Vancouver, it came as a surprise when, on April 11, I received an email from Samantha Giordano, asking that we please remove her headshot and bio from AIM's website. She had voiced an early concern that some would deem our newly launched program as a competitive fundraising campaign versus UAB, but never imagined the lengths that would be used to derail our efforts. Unfortunately, Samantha had been contacted by her supervisor and was afraid that she would not graduate if her information remained on our "About Us" page. It was extremely hard to see Samantha go, but I respected her immensely and didn't want to compromise her education and future in any way.

The following day, upon Candace's return from Canada, she called me into her office and claimed that my activities with AIM were in violation of UAB's conflict of interest policy, the conflict of commitment policy, and the external activity policy. Therefore, she instructed me to stop all activities with AIM while I was an employee at UAB.

I nearly had a heart attack standing in her office. I had had no warning or hint that Candace was upset with my involvement with AIM. In fact, I believed we were on even better terms, as we had discussed ways in which her laboratory and AIM might collaborate and that, hopefully, her laboratory would receive funding from our new grant program.

I paused for several minutes, searching my brain for anything I had missed that could possibly justify her anger-filled accusations. AIM a "conflict of interest." How? In what way? And most importantly, why would AIM be considered a conflict if we were trying to raise funds for scientific research at the university? The logic was unclear, but it crossed my mind that perhaps she was resentful of our goals to build a research program outside the walls of UAB. Other thoughts raced through my head, but before I could make sense of any of them, Candace told me that I would not be allowed to come back to my office again if I was going to pursue activities with AIM. I shook my head in disbelief and explained that there must have been a misunderstanding pertaining to my employment, as she was aware that I had put in my letter of resignation, with the proper thirty-day notice, dated April 8, 2013. My last day of employment should be May 10, 2013, still another month away. I also reminded her that I had requested a personal day to participate in a press conference for AIM on April 18, which had already been approved by her on several different occasions. I even had text messages on my phone that showed she had approved my day off from work.

Her temper flared with each word, so I took an early lunch and called AIM's legal counselor, Kathryn Gentle, for advice. Kathryn advised me to return to work and continue with my responsibilities until May 10, unless otherwise notified by Candace or UAB's Human Resources Department.

It was a typical bumper-to-bumper drive home in five o'clock traffic on Highway 280, allowing me plenty of time to fill Ron in on my unbelievable day with Candace. He stopped by our home after his last hip replacement case for the day and did a wonderful job of distracting my thoughts away from work by watching a fun movie with the children and me. Suddenly, out of the corner of his eye, he noticed movement—a shadow change—on the front porch. Having had two decades of paramilitary background experience with a high threat protection group called Triple Canopy, Ron knew this was not a tree limb moving in the wind, nor a cloud streaking across the moon. As the odd shadow turned into a silhouette of a tall man, Ron was certain this was not a common thief trying to case our house. Observing him standing frozen like an ice sculpture to blend into the column on our porch, Ron knew this was a professional, dressed in military blackout gear, who was trained and on a mission.

Without alarming the children, me, or the intruder, Ron slowly stood up from the couch and walked in the opposite direction, away from the front of my home. He eased out the back door, circled around the east side of the house with his hand gripping his pocket knife, and followed a row of boxwood shrubs that led to the front porch. In an attempt to flank the intruder, Ron crouched down and sprinted across the yard; however, before he could make it over a brick retaining wall along the driveway, the intruder darted across the street and fled between two homes, disappearing into the darkness. After the police arrived, Ron gave a full description of the intruder, along with details of the escape route used.

The police told us that this episode appeared to be a preplanned attack or a home invasion. I was deeply shaken to say the least. But why? I tried to think. It was impossible, even with the recent unpleasantness at work, that the incident might be related to my involvement with AIM. *Who would do this? Was this a scare tactic to distract me from my activities with stem cell research?*

The next morning, Ron called a friend from Triple Canopy and arranged for a representative to fly to Birmingham and sit down with us and review the situation. In their assessment, Triple Canopy would provide realistic measures of what was needed to ensure our safety and security. These measures could range anywhere from little things that my children and I could do, all the way up to providing actual security personnel to protect our family.

Two days later, Roman flew back to Alabama and helped me to sort through everything AIM related. On April 18, we officially launched the Alabama Institute of Medicine by hosting a press conference at the Disability Rights and Resource Center in downtown Birmingham. With heavy security on the premises, TJ and his family arrived first, followed by Dr. Wick and Dr. Murphy-Ullrich of UAB, Graham Sisson of the Governor's Office on Disability, Dr. Raj Singh, who served as AIM's external scientific advisor and CEO of Vivo Biosciences, Inc., and Yann Ranaivo of the *Birmingham Business Journal*. After the successful press event, Roman and I found it odd that Candace claimed AIM was a conflict of interest to UAB, yet two high-ranking faculty members had participated in our event and publicly acknowledged their support of our research grant program. *What were we missing?* I asked myself over and over again.

The most extreme encounter with Candace took place the next morning on April 19, when my personal belongings were boxed up and removed from my office at UAB and delivered to the benefit golf tournament I had organized to help support TJ's spinal cord injury program at the Department of Physical Medicine and Rehabilitation. Under my leadership of the event and with the help of other foundation board members, the golf tournament raised over $24,000, which left many volunteers and supporters questioning why my hard work had gone unrecognized and unappreciated by Candace. Her behavior seemed capricious, small, and undeserved.

I was feeling completely devastated, and it could have been so easy for me to turn away from my dreams of helping others through AIM. But there was no way I was giving up. Instead, I embraced this new season of spring when the days quietly lengthen and the beautiful blooms spread their message of hope across the earth. More determined than ever, I decided to let hope drive me too. Not only was I going to build AIM into the great stem cell institute of the southeast we envisioned, but also I was not going to let any individual or group prevent AIM from achieving its purpose.

20

ONWARDS AND UPWARDS

Alabama and California
April–October 2013

The morning after the golf tournament, I called Kathryn Gentle and made an appointment with her for the following Monday. She was concerned that our efforts with AIM were being sabotaged and was prepared to take stronger, legal actions if necessary. Because her expertise was in nonprofits and family law, she consulted with an employment law attorney who believed that I could have several claims, including wrongful termination and tortious interference, with the business relations of AIM. Instead of becoming distracted with a major lawsuit, I remained on high alert for suspicious activity but focused solely on our goals and objectives for AIM.

And so for the remainder of April and early May, I began recruiting volunteers, members to AIM's board of directors, and staff. TJ was top on our list for board membership, and we also hoped he would serve in an administrative role on our grant program. On May 10, I attended his graduation from nursing school in Mobile and asked if he would consider joining our team. A week later, TJ confirmed his membership, and accepted the position as patient advocate coordinator of AIM. He also told us he was very interested and willing to relocate to Birmingham if the financials were right for his move. So with Roman's help to cover his immediate expenses, on May 22, TJ moved into a two-bedroom apartment just fifteen minutes away from downtown Birmingham.

It was a complete joy having TJ in Birmingham. My children were ecstatic and felt like family was finally nearby. Ron enjoyed his company just as much and built a wheelchair ramp at his home so that TJ could visit anytime. TJ and I jumped immediately into work for AIM and accomplished more than I could have imagined. We planned fundraising events, solicited sponsors, and began our education program by sharing our AIM-4-Cure message with anyone who would listen, including local television and radio stations, newspapers and magazines, and disability advocacy groups. Our efforts gave us great confidence that the three-part strategy for AIM we had envisioned six months before was attainable and achievable.

The first phase of our plan consisted of a granting program. Scientists would go through a request for application (RFA) process for funding in support of their stem cell research of any disease, injury, or field of ailment. We anticipated only a handful of applications for our first round of funding, which we hoped to announce the following spring. We also believed the requested range of funding would be between $100,000 and $300,000 or more for "proof of concept"—proof the idea scientifically works—in the laboratory. When projects are successful and move beyond the pilot-study phase and into human clinical trials, funding typically ranges well into the eight-figure amounts. AIM hoped to begin by funding several pilot studies with 90 percent of all donations being directly deposited into AIM's Scientific Research Grant Trust account.

Early on, we realized that we needed a state-of-the-art, privately funded laboratory where researchers could check politics at the door and do the most advanced and sophisticated stem cell work in-house. In the second phase of our program, AIM would build a core laboratory in Jefferson County, where qualified scientists from all over Alabama could use AIM's cutting-edge equipment, space, and scientific experience.

Finally, phase three of our plan would develop hospital space where regenerative medicine treatments could be administered and where patients suffering from chronic disease, injury, or ailment could receive on-site treatment in Alabama.

Each phase of the Alabama Institute of Medicine would move a step closer to offering the most advanced therapies and cures for our state, and the world. AIM's planning committee, staff, and board of directors could not know how many years it would take us to accomplish these goals, but we were determined to persevere and get through each phase and beyond!

To help us develop phase one, we turned to Dr. Raj Singh of Vivo Biosciences, Inc. (VBI), a Birmingham biotech company established in 2004 and based on technology Raj developed while working as a pathology professor at UAB. Vivo Biosciences' flagship product, HuBiogel, acted as a glue for cells. Raj owned the only world patent for this 3-D human matrix, which was clinical grade and used for tissue regeneration. At VBI, Raj used HuBiogel to develop tumor models that cancer drugs could be tested on.

Raj recommended we strengthen our relationships with local institutions, so TJ thought it would be beneficial for our group to discuss possible collaborations with Candace at UAB. I, too, felt a relationship with Candace should be nurtured, and so I encouraged TJ to set up a meeting with my former boss. On June 7, he emailed this message to Candace and Raj with me cc'd:

> Hi Dr. Singh and Dr. Floyd,
>
> Ms. Tory and I have a meeting at 11 a.m. on Monday so we are going to try and figure out a good time and date next week when we are all free. Is there another time when either of you are available on Monday? If not we will set it up for another day next week if possible.
>
> I look forward to hearing from both of you. Thank you all so much as I feel that it is my privilege to set this meeting up.
>
> Best Regards,
>
> TJ Atchison
> Patient Advocate Coordinator, AIM
> www.aim4cure.org

Raj responded that Tuesday at 1 p.m. worked best for him. I waited nervously for Candace's response, as my last encounter with her at the golf tournament was a complete disaster when she had my office belongings literally dumped into Ron's truck. She also made every possible effort to fluster me in front of the tournament's volunteers and attendees and never once acknowledged the effort I had put into making this event a success for her laboratory.

Surprisingly, she responded and confirmed her availability for the following Tuesday.

TJ and I met Raj in the lobby of the Spain Rehabilitation Center. Sensing my nervousness, Raj reassured me that everything would go smoothly during our meeting. His encouraging words helped me to relax, but there was a lingering feeling that the outcome with Candace would not be collaborative. Keeping a slow pace, Raj led us inside to my former office, which was now occupied by a young lady whom I recognized as another UAB administrative assistant. I didn't know her that well and had only bumped into her a few times in passing from our department head's office downstairs. Our eyes met, and the look of sadness and stress across her face made me eternally grateful that my goals for AIM had taken me down a different path.

I felt safe sitting between Raj and TJ at the conference table and did my best to remain calm throughout the meeting. It was only minutes into Raj's presentation that I became frustrated with Candace's observations regarding his technology and data. Raj was a brilliant researcher and inventor and had achieved more accolades in his career than many researchers in the state. I sensed Candace's sharp-edged comments stemmed from the fact that she had never been a champion of human embryonic stem cells, as her primary focus for spinal cord injury repair included the use of Schwann cells—a type of adult cell found throughout the entire peripheral nervous system (PNS). The PNS includes all nerves going out to muscles as well as sensory nerves coming from the muscles back to the spinal cord. Schwann cells produce the myelin for sensory and motor axons only of the PNS, and can wrap around only one axon at a time. As a coinvestigator on the study that was published in the *Journal of Neurochemistry*, November 2010, Candace and her colleagues reported: "Schwann cell transplantation is a promising repair strategy after spinal cord injury; however, a large number of Schwann cells do not survive following transplantation."

Keeping his professional composure, Raj disregarded Candace's comments and finished his presentation about the promise of combining his HuBiogel technology with embryonic stem cells and Schwann cells in the repair of spinal cord injury. Raj believed his HuBiogel was the missing link, and if combined with any stem cell type, this would allow their survival following transplantation. TJ and I sat quietly at the table, our faces betraying no emotion one way or the other. We jotted down notes and occasionally nodded our heads, showing Dr. Singh we were listening carefully as he presented to Candace.

As soon as Raj completed his talk, Candace stood from the table and looked me in the eyes. With her face flushing, she asked in an arrogant tone, "Why is she in this meeting?"

Yes, the "she" meant me.

More confused than ever, I turned to Raj and TJ and waited for one of them to respond.

TJ dropped his head, took a deep breath, then said, "Ms. Tory is here because I asked her to join us in discussion of a potential study for treatment of spinal cord injury."

Candace said, "I have made it very clear that AIM is a conflict of interest to UAB, and I will not be associated with any activities related to this organization."

TJ attempted to clarify my presence by saying, "But AIM wants to fund a study for spinal cord injury, and I'd like to use the core laboratory here at UAB to perform the animal studies. I am sure there's a way we can work this out."

Candace angrily threw her pen across the table. "I will not discuss anything more if she stays in this meeting."

At this point, I was completely humiliated and felt embarrassed for TJ, Raj, and for myself.

In a tearful voice, I said, "Candace, I do not understand what is going on. I am here to help fund this study and your research. If we work together on this project, there is potential that better treatment, or perhaps a cure, for spinal cord injury can result."

She laughed. "You know exactly what is going on here, Tory. I'm through with this conversation."

In an effort to avoid further abuse to myself or the group, my eyes beginning to water, I gathered my purse and writing tools and excused myself from the meeting. Raj shook his head in disbelief and followed me outside. We made our way down the hallway and found it odd that TJ stayed behind in Candace's office. I heard the door close behind but did not look back. I only assumed that he was asking her to please show professionalism during future meetings, but unfortunately, as I was to learn, this was not the case. It would take several weeks before I pieced together what had actually transpired during TJ's and Candace's closed-door conversation.

Two days later, TJ and I met at Raj's office in Five Points—the business, dining, and entertainment district of Birmingham—to tour the 6,000-square-foot Vivo Biosciences research facility. No one mentioned that terrible meeting with Candace; instead we brainstormed ways to collaborate with researchers on the West Coast. I emailed my friend Michelle at UC-Irvine and arranged for Dr. Singh to travel to California to meet with stem cell pioneer Dr. Hans Keirstead. Roman and I believed it would be remarkable to combine Dr. Singh's HuBiogel with Dr. Keirstead's stem cells.

And so on June 26, 2013, TJ, Raj, and I flew to UC-Irvine and met with Dr. Keirstead. During our flight from Atlanta to California, I updated Raj and TJ on the progress of Hans's research since his collaboration with Geron had ended in 2010. Hans had advanced a melanoma study into human clinical trials and was wrapping up a Phase 1 safety trial for a liver cancer treatment in China. He was moving rapidly toward a Phase 2 trial, in the United States, of a treatment for ovarian cancer and was also contemplating whether to transition his privately owned company, California Stem Cell, Inc., into a publicly traded company. It was no surprise that Hans had been offered over $700 million from angel investors to remain a private company, but he was certainly entertaining the idea of going public in order to move these studies, along with filing a new FDA application for ovarian cancer, toward human clinical trials.

I was thrilled to introduce TJ and Raj to Hans, who seemed overwhelmed to finally meet his first patient injected with GRNOPC1. Hans was impressed by our success in launching AIM and was moved by our mission and strategic plan. I further explained that AIM's top priority was to raise over $1 million before next spring and to begin funding studies no later than August 2014. Hans was well aware that, because AIM was declared a privately funded organization under the IRS, our research program could take on high-risk projects (both controversial and very early science studies that had little data to demonstrate effectiveness) that would normally not receive public funding or consideration.

Wanting our program to succeed more than anything, Hans offered to serve as an external scientific advisor for our program and also to donate any line of his stem cells in collaboration with projects Roman and I recommended through AIM. This excited Dr. Singh, because he was very interested in testing his HuBiogel matrix with Hans's stem cells, specifically his neuronal progenitor cells. These self-renewal cells reside in the adult nervous system and help maintain the brain and spinal cord. Dr. Singh's and Dr. Keirstead's technologies were unique for many reasons, mainly because both had received excellent peer reviews and FDA approval for their work, and both of their respective methods and technologies were commercially developed and available for mass market distribution. Advanced cells with an advanced delivery system would be an optimal project for angel investors or a research program like AIM to consider funding. I could not wait to share this exciting news with Roman.

Just two days later, Roman met TJ, Raj, and me in San Francisco and arranged for us to tour the Gladstone Institute. Roman's great friend and director of the Gladstone Institute, Dr. Deepak Srivastava, invited us inside the laboratory of Nobel Prize winner Shinya Yamanaka. This was such an amazing experience, to see where the researcher had produced the world's first human induced pluripotent stem (IPS) cells and discovered that mature cells could be reprogrammed to become pluripotent, meaning these cells could become all cell types in the adult body. Our visit with Dr. Srivastava ended with a closed-door conversation about his potential collaboration with researchers back in Alabama, including Raj.

The following day, we took a cab to the airport for our departure flights. Raj was tremendously excited by the opportunities that had come out of our California trip. He and I agreed to meet the following week in Birmingham to regroup and determine which projects to pursue. I had a hunch we would move forward with Hans first, as he seemed most eager to collaborate with Raj.

Raj and TJ gave me a quick hug good-bye, and then we headed to different terminals for our departure flights. TJ was returning to Birmingham while Raj was en route to North Carolina for another round of biotech meetings through the weekend. As for my destination, I was thrilled to be heading to San Francisco, where Ron had planned a romantic getaway for us while our children spent the weekend with family back home.

Ron and I found ourselves in one of the most beautiful spots in the world—Napa, California. At the Carneros Inn, on top of a hill at their most gorgeous viewpoint, we were sitting in white Adirondack chairs, taking pictures of ourselves with the hills, wide as angels' wings, as our backdrop. Ron took his phone and started a panoramic video. He smiled like a teenager preparing for prom as he announced, "This is a moment we will cherish forever." He stood and took my hand, then got down on one knee and pulled a ring box from his pocket. It was June 28, my mother's birthday, when Ron proposed against a glittering sky. It was absolutely the most perfect setting. I was truly surprised and happily said, "YES!"

We spent our final evening in California wrapped in each other's arms and taking in the peace and tranquility that came with no work, no children, and no deadlines. It was heaven. In fact, this down time was exactly what Ron and I needed to charge up for our next year of advocacy, fundraising, and advancing the biotech industry in Alabama.

Five weeks later, our lives were formally joined. Ron's close friend and preacher Matt Scott performed the ceremony at the Vestavia Country Club. As we were pronounced husband and wife, I looked into Ron's sweet face and told him that I would love him forever. He had my heart and it felt amazing to know that we were blessed with each other and our beautiful children for as long as we lived.

The weekend after our marriage, with a honeymoon on hold until our schedules settled down, Ron and I spent hours and hours unloading boxes from storage and from my home in Liberty Park into his 1970s A-frame home built of dark stones and wood-paneled walls. Ron had chosen this home for its breathtaking views of the rolling hills, which gave him a feeling of peace and contentment with life and with nature.

Unpacking our last load from storage, Ron and I laughed, as we had no idea where we were going to possibly put everything, children included. Our neighbors and friends teased us, calling us the "Brady Bunch Family!" And rightly so, there were nine of us, including seven children from the ages of seventeen to six years old. Indeed, our hearts were filled with happiness, and most importantly, the comfort of having a loving family.

Back at AIM headquarters, aka Raj's conference room at Vivo Biosciences, Roman joined us by Skype for a teleconference with our corporate attorney, who helped us form a company called VivoStem, LLC. The goal of our new company would be to create unique intellectual properties by combining Raj's HuBiogel matrix with stem cell therapies from top researchers like Hans and Deepak Srivastava of California and others across the globe. We would be extremely selective in our partnerships and only collaborate with those researchers who owned patents for stem cell applications that held the promise of potential remedies for spinal cord injuries, diabetes, cardiac disease, cancer, sports injury, and wound healing. We were eager to collaborate with Hans, so the recommended approach by our legal counsel was to establish this company first, and then combine technologies so we didn't have to duplicate or reinvent the wheel for each application of our portfolio. It was a wise decision to establish VivoStem before signing business contracts with Hans or other researchers, so that when these term agreements were finalized approximately three to six months later, our company would demonstrate significant growth and value. Then we would work aggressively to attract shareholder interest and validate our goal of becoming a leading biotech company by 2016.

Despite the progress being made with both AIM and VivoStem, TJ felt his program at UAB was suffering from his involvement with AIM, so he turned in his letter of resignation on August 18, telling us he had decided to focus all of his time and energy on supporting Candace's research at UAB. To some degree, I understood TJ's decision because I knew how crucial maintaining those relationships at the university and at the state capital were to ensuring TJ's Law remained included in the Education Trust Fund budget. His role as spokesperson for the spinal cord injury program was very demanding and required more hours than he first imagined. But his lack of emotion or concern for AIM's progress made me wonder if his decision to resign from AIM and halt his advocacy for human embryonic stem cell research had been influenced by Candace, who I assumed remained angry with us.

During the next several months, Roman, Raj, Hans, and I moved forward with VivoStem. We exchanged memoranda of understanding (MOU) and provided financial statements, along with patent information to determine the working budget we would need for beginning an animal trial. Chief among our list of projects was the combination of neuronal progenitor cells and HuBiogel. We wanted to see if these cellular components could be used together, in tandem, to form an effective repair for damaged spinal cord tissue. Our legal counsel and company accountant suggested that if funds were available to complete animal studies, VivoStem, LLC, could see positive results and be fully functional as early as spring 2015. Not only did this projection give hope of funding additional projects, but it also held significant potential to change the field of medicine by combining the perfect delivery system with the highly sought after stem cell line belonging to our great ally Dr. Hans

Keirstead. But the projections kept getting better, as our accountant indicated that VivoStem's current value was at $1.5 million, with the potential to increase to $20 million before 2017. He also explained that we would be able to donate a high percentage of VivoStem's capital back into AIM if we determined to do so.

Roman, Raj, and I agreed that we would pledge the maximum amount allowed of our net profits from VivoStem, and from joint publications, to help fund research projects. This was wonderful news, and provided assurance that AIM would, indeed, have a stable flow of funding from our new ventures.

Not only were the projections looking favorable for VivoStem, but AIM was also gaining momentum as we welcomed cooler weather and another great year of Southeastern Conference (SEC) football by hosting two major fundraising events in succession during September and October. We held our inaugural Workplay Gala fundraising dinner on September 26, 2013, at the beautiful Workplay Ballroom in downtown Birmingham. The well-attended event promoted funding for AIM research, grants, and scholarships across the state and featured local musical artist Sarah Simmons, a finalist on the 2013 season of NBC's *The Voice*. Dr. Joanne Murphy-Ullrich of UAB's BERM Center spoke to the crowd of the importance of regenerative medicine and its integral role in contributing to the future of health care. She was a very wise and inspirational speaker, and we were fortunate to have her attend our Gala and speak on behalf of UAB/AIM collaborations.

Our second event, Tailgate for Cure, featured multiple big screens showing SEC football throughout the day and a live radio remote from WJOX. Taylor Hicks headlined the concert, which included other musical performances by Sarah Simmons; Tim Hockenberry, a San Francisco–based artist and *America's Got Talent* semifinalist; and the band Within Reason, winner of the 2013 Grammy Awards' Gig of a Lifetime. Fans had the opportunity to meet these artists as well as former football athletes Marquis Maze, Brandon Gibson, Tyronne King, and Kareem McNeal. Various activities inside the Kid Zone kept children of all ages entertained throughout the day.

"It's because of programs like the Alabama Institute of Medicine that all people in our state and across the world will have the opportunity to receive advanced medical treatments and hopefully receive cures for disease and injury," stated Birmingham native and *American Idol* winner Taylor Hicks.

The event came to a close around 11 p.m. with fans, musicians, celebrities, and our volunteers having a deeper understanding of AIM's mission and goals. But even more important, they learned that medical breakthroughs of the scale imagined depended on events like these and many others that we were planning for the future.

21

CONNECT–COLLABORATE–CURE

New York, New York, and Birmingham, Alabama
October 2013–June 2014

October came to an end with enthusiasm and support gathered for our research program. As part of our rollout with AIM, it seemed like a good time to make another run with "The Human Candidate." I had a new literary agent now, who, like Mac, requested that I secure letters of support from both key people in the story and from leading experts in the stem cell community. A work trip to New York unrelated to the book was planned for the end of the month, but we decided that while I was there, I would try to see a few book editors and present my repositioned text along with an update on our recent successes. I discovered, however, I was naive to believe the letter I needed most—TJ's—would come easily.

Since my last encounter with Candace in June, during our meeting with Raj and TJ to discuss possible AIM funding for her research laboratory, I realized the hard way that her closed-door conversation with TJ was far more treacherous than what I assumed was a pep talk by him encouraging professionalism with members of our group.

On October 24, TJ emailed me requesting my help in sending him a photo that I'd had on file since my days as educational liaison and program manager of his spinal cord injury program at UAB. I located the image and attached it to my own request:

> Dear TJ,
>
> Attached is the TJAF Logo in jpeg format. I'm also reaching out to you today to ask for your help by writing a letter of support on my behalf for upcoming meetings with patient advocacy groups and editors in New York.
>
> If you could please reply with your personal letter no later than Tuesday, October 29th, I would be very grateful. Please let me know if you have any questions or feedback.
>
> Thank you in advance for your help with this request. Moving mountains for our cures, always! Sending my very best, and continued prayers for you and your job search in Mobile.
>
> All best,
> Tory Williams

TJ texted me that evening to say that he was traveling but would take a close look at my note as soon as possible. Three days passed without hearing from him, so I sent a friendly text reminding him that I needed the letter of support by week's end if possible. He was quick to respond that he found my email buried in a pile and would work on the letter over the weekend. On October 30, I received this text from TJ:

> I am planning on writing the letter. It's the least I can do. I'm just trying to figure out how to not get my program in bad blood with UAB. I was wondering if I could write it and send it directly to all of the groups and individuals you wanted to have it? This way the letter is from me personally which should mean more to the groups I would think. Is that a problem?

My response:

> I would feel more comfortable including it in the portfolio package with all the other letters of support. This will also give you plausible deniability if anyone from any organization has an issue with you showing me personal support. As long as it's not on UAB letterhead, you are writing this letter of support as a family friend, a relationship which we have both acknowledged hundreds of times. No organization or individual can dictate who

> you support on a personal level. If they indicate otherwise, they are in the wrong!

Five minutes later, this is the text I received:

> Hey, I think at this time it would not be good for me to write the letter of support for you because of the confusion people still have differentiating between my research program and AIM. I think UAB would frown upon my research program if they see that a letter of support to you was written in my name. I guess if I changed the name of my research program, and Law, then this might resolve most of the issues we're currently facing. If it would help, you could even call me during each of your meetings so that whoever you're meeting with can hear me state my gratitude for the work that you've done and are currently doing in the fight to cure chronic illness.

His response made very little sense to me. Why would anyone frown upon his personal support for a project that we had been working on for nearly two years before passing TJ's Law? I had made great friends at the university and considered our organizations to be partners in this fight for cures. This didn't add up in my mind, and it certainly didn't sound like the same TJ I had worked so closely with to pass a law in his name, charter a new state program, and raise thousands of dollars to help find a cure for his disability—and the young man I had grown to love like a brother.

My response was one of utter shock and disbelief. With my fingers trembling, I typed the only word that came to mind, "Unbelievable . . ."

TJ followed up with, "I hope you know I do want it to be known that you have my support."

Seeing one face in particular pass through my mind, I asked, "Who is advising you?"

And then there was no response on his end.

The only thing I took away from that stinging thread was a broken heart and a feeling of despair for everything I had done for TJ and his program.

That night, Ron held me tightly and stroked his fingers through my hair as I cried myself to sleep. The next morning, I could not focus on anything. As snippets of the last three years played over and over inside my head like a bad movie, all I could think about was how much I had risked and given up to help TJ and Candace. Ron couldn't make sense of these recent text messages either, and felt we should seek legal advice.

But I had no more steam in my engine and didn't want this web of disappointments to tighten any further. Then at the perfect moment, my youngest daughter Courtney kneeled next to me and pulled me out of this darkness with her sweet words: "Mommy, I don't know what monster crawled into your bed, but you've got to get yourself together today!"

I had to laugh and hugged Courtney close. Her comment reminded me that I had so much to feel grateful for, and that I could not move forward if I did not find closure regarding these recent events. I drove to my parents' home for the weekend and spent hours talking with my mother at our favorite spot—the front porch. She helped me realize that even when someone goes into something with the best intentions and purest of heart, things happen. Colleagues don't always work collaboratively. A better offer comes along and someone leaves, leaving a great hole, but also creating new opportunities for fresh ideas. People become frustrated by the slow pace of progress, the bureaucracy around getting anything done, risk-aversion, poor decision-making, leadership changes, changes in vision and focus. And research laboratories, even the best ones that are doing science in the cause of humanity, are managed by . . . humans.

Later that week, I received a message from my friend Anita, who naturally supported her son and let me know that, by extension, she supported Candace. Anita asked why I felt so "threatened" by Candace and said that I should just stay out of the picture so her research could move forward. I didn't have the heart to tell Anita what had occurred during my employment at TJ's spinal cord program because I was afraid the truth would push her and TJ away from the program and for advocating for these important cures. Ultimately, our friendship became strained and finally there was nothing more I could do, no words I could say, but to wish them well and to keep the door open if they ever wanted to reach out.

For Roman, myself, and the millions of others suffering from disease and injury, I swallowed my disappointment and embraced a tentative, tumbled wisdom. I would not give up on AIM or my desire to help others. But I could only control what was in front of me, and this was my family's well-being, my writing projects, my friendships, and my altruistic purpose of making a difference in the lives of the people around me. So I decided to use my gift of moving through terrible situations by taking the first step forward and focusing on the positives in my life.

Ron was a constant source of strength and support and convinced me that the trip to New York was a much-needed getaway for us both. So instead of meeting with book editors, I focused my attention on the meetings I'd planned with researchers and with administrators at the New York Stem Cell Foundation. David McKeon, chief of staff of the New York Stem Cell Foundation, for instance, was most incredible, and helped me develop important AIM research collaborations with the NYSF. He also offered to connect me with the legendary Bernard Siegel, founder and executive director of the Genetics Policy Institute.

From my research, I knew Mr. Siegel first became involved with the scientific community in 2002, when he filed a landmark case seeking a guardian for the alleged human clone, "Baby Eve." The case was widely credited for exposing Clonaid, the "human cloning company" as a sham. More important, it initiated conversations between scientists and policy experts nationwide about the need for legal and policy advocates for the scientific community. In 2003, Mr. Siegel founded the Genetics Policy Institute, where he has continued to do pioneering advocacy work on behalf of patients, doctors, and researchers involved with the regenerative medicine community.

I greatly appreciated David's generosity and this email to Mr. Siegel on my behalf:

> Dear Bernie,
>
> I met yesterday with Tory Williams who has started a non-profit called the Alabama Institute of Medicine (AIM). You may remember Tory as she was working with TJ Atchison (the first patient to participate in Geron's clinical trial). She has done a lot of work in advocating for stem cell research and has even been successful in passing legislation in Alabama that results in $400,000 a year going to spinal cord injury research at UAB.
>
> As Tory is just getting up and started, I thought that you would be a great person for her to meet with. Tory is a patient advocate and I couldn't think of a better patient advocate to connect her with. She is working with a number of people you know such as Roman Reed who is the Chairman of AIM's Board of Directors and Hans Keirstead who is Chairman of AIM's External Scientific Advisory Board. I thought it would be great for Tory to speak or meet with you either at the World Stem Cell Summit or in Florida. I hope the two of you can connect!
>
> Best,
> David

David's kindness, coming as it did at a time when I was feeling so bruised, was an energy shot for the advancement of AIM. His actions renewed my faith in people's inherent goodness and that most do not need a "return of investment" to do a good deed for another. David simply wanted to help a good cause. I will forever be grateful to him. And, in fact, Bernie responded within an hour of David's email suggesting we get together while at the World Stem Cell Summit in San Diego a few weeks later.

The WSCS sounded like an important event to attend, but our finances were slim, as I was not receiving a salary from AIM. Roman and I had decided to forgo compensation until after AIM had reached $1 million in the research grant account, while Ron was entangled in various business matters regarding patent infringement on his CABLZ eyewear retainer system. But we knew how important the World Stem Cell Summit meeting could be for networking and attracting donors to AIM, and so we decided to take the risk. On December 3, my mother drove to Birmingham to babysit our children while we attended the WSCS. After a quick hug of appreciation to Mom for making herself available to babysit, Ron and I, along with two AIM supporters, all traveling at our own expense, flew to San Diego with the shared goal of advancing stem cell research in Alabama.

Roman met us at the WSCS registration table and embraced Ron and me with hugs and words of appreciation for making the trip. It was a pleasure to introduce Roman to our group, which included Chris Drummond, a young private equity investor who had learned business and finance from his father, Garry Neil Drummond, CEO of Drummond Company, a global leader in coal production and, according to the Forbes list, one of America's largest private companies.

Another member of our group was Chris's friend Raleigh Kent, who learned the complexities of the medical industry from his father, Dr. Raleigh Kent, a well-respected and highly successful Birmingham surgeon. Raleigh had worked with Ron at Stryker Orthopaedics for over five years and was a shareholder with Chris and Ron in another venture, a spin-off company of AIM called Wellpace Medical, LLC, located in Birmingham. Wellpace's mission was to distribute stem cell and other medical products to cosmetic stores, pharmacies, hospital buying groups, and doctors at a competitive rate.

The momentum and positive energy from this three-day event carried over into our return trip to Alabama. Through the World Stem Cell

Summit and meeting Bernie Siegel and his team at Genetics Policy Institute, AIM was able to share the advances we were making in the stem cell community and express our interest to host the World Stem Cell Summit in Alabama in the years to come.

Chris was particularly encouraged by the issues addressed during the event, which featured more than 150 speakers and fifty hours of in-depth presentations, all pertinent to translating basic research into cures, and included discussions on the latest scientific discoveries, business models, legal and regulatory solutions, and best practices. After learning more about research reimbursements, financing, venture capital, and economic development, Chris felt encouraged to support AIM's entry into this biotech ecosystem. He believed AIM had the potential to one day become a leader in the field and felt his financial contribution could truly make a difference for a start-up program like AIM, and in the lives of millions.

So after our return trip to Alabama, and several coffee shop meetings, group teleconferences, and email exchanges later, this incredible supporter became a benefactor and made a generous $1 million gift to AIM to advance stem cell research in Alabama. After sharing the wonderful news with AIM's board of directors, we officially announced this significant milestone for our program. Very modestly, Chris asked us not to disclose his name as the benefactor in hopes that the focus would remain on the research and not on his donation, which we gratefully did.

Chris's commitment to AIM was a natural one because our progressive research interested him, and our program supported the creation of jobs that he hoped would keep talented researchers in our state. His wish was that his donation would inspire many others to make similar contributions to our groundbreaking organization. And in fact, we saw an uptick in donations to AIM, with checks pouring in not just from Alabama, but also from benefactors across the country. The range was between twenty-five dollars to several thousand—each one important and necessary in moving the dial.

With Chris's donation, we were most eager to begin our granting process, so we rallied our legal team, our accounting department, and formed our Scientific Review Committee, which was led by the researcher and biotech administrator, Dr. Jane Lebkowski, who had served as VP of regenerative medicine and chief scientific officer at Geron Corporation during development and launch of the GRNOPC1 clinical trial.

In 2010, when Dr. Lebkowski and many other top executives left Geron, including its medical director, Edward Wirth, they established a new partnership through Asterias Biotherapeutics (a subsidiary of BioTime) and bought the stem cell properties from Geron to resume the spinal cord injury trials.

During our early efforts to establish AIM, Dr. Lebkowski was one of the first researchers that Roman and I contacted in hopes she would join our team in some capacity. With their long friendship, Dr. Lebkowski was quick to jump on board and help Roman and our nonprofit. We also brought Melissa King on to AIM's board of directors. As program director for operations and communications for the California Research and Cures Coalition, Melissa had been an instrumental member of the team that successfully advocated for the passage of Proposition 71 in November 2004. She also served for six years as executive director of CIRM's governing board.

With the hoped-for funds now in the research grant account and an incredible team of directors leading our efforts, Roman and I wasted no time in emailing Jane announcing that we were ready to open our doors for business. Jane patiently walked us through the process of posting our application online and establishing the guidelines for our granting process. With AIM's board of directors' guidance, we set a deadline date of May 21 for all research proposals to be submitted to AIM's Scientific Grant Review Committee. Our team was thrilled to receive a total of eight applications, more than we dared to anticipate for a start-up like ours. All of the proposals contained interesting ideas and included novel stem cell components, which validated our belief that many researchers in Alabama were in need of a program like AIM to fund their stem cell projects.

Just nine days later, on May 30, 2014, Jane received important news as well. Her company, Asterias, had been approved for $14.3 million from the California Institute of Medicine (CIRM) for the spinal cord injury project application (formerly the Geron trial study) submitted six months earlier. This funding, which we all deeply hope will bring human embryonic stem cell treatment closer to paralyzed people, helped close a great circle in my journey to share this story by bringing scientists, biotech industry, patients, and advocates together, united in strength and perseverance for cures—and surely, the dream of a public and private partnership being demonstrated as a working reality.

Back in Alabama, we were happy to share the news of Asterias' resuming the Geron trials with our friends, supporters, and all who had interest in the stem cell research field. I wanted badly to reach out to TJ and offer him encouragement and hope that research was moving forward. But after several hours of deliberation and staring at his cell number pulled up on my dial-pad, I decided it was best to leave things as they were to avoid any negative issues resurfacing for us. Instead of calling or texting TJ, I hoped he would notice the links to this wonderful news posted on my personal Facebook page, where we remained "friends."

Meanwhile, Dr. Lebkowski and her committee worked diligently to review the eight research proposals submitted to AIM. She and her team spent nearly a month reviewing these applications, and made their official recommendations three days ahead of our deadline. In her final notes, she confirmed that the process had been double-blinded, and that the grantee did not know the reviewers, and the reviewers did not know the grantee, so that there would be no conflicts of interests issues.

On June 17, AIM's board of directors voted and approved three research grants totaling near $1 million. One project grant went to Thomas Ryan, PhD, and his team at the University of Alabama at Birmingham (UAB) to extend by four years the preclinical studies of gene editing as a treatment for sickle cell anemia and Cooley's anemia, a study that, if successful, would demonstrate safe and effective treatments of many more hematopoietic disorders. This grant would fund $750,000 distributed over four years, contingent on the study team meeting research milestones during the first two years of the project.

The second grant was for Palaniappan Sethu, PhD, and his lab at UAB to further his work in using a cardiac cell culture model to provide appropriate mechanical stresses on cultured cardiomyocytes to facilitate and accelerate their maturation. They proposed that such a system could be used to "precondition" pluripotent stem cell–derived cardiomyocytes prior to their transplantation into the heart to facilitate their survival and integration into the diseased heart. This grant would fund $100,000 for year one, with AIM's board of directors revisiting the proposal in year two to determine whether research milestones had been achieved, in which case a second year of funding would be approved at another $100,000.

The third grant was awarded to Kejin Hu, PhD, and his team at UAB to study the roles of the human PODXL gene in human embryonic stem cells (hESC) and induced pluripotent stem (IPS) cells. The proposed work was focused on preliminary characterization of the function of the PODXL gene, especially as it relates to creation and maintenance of the pluripotent state in pluripotent stem cells. This grant would fund $100,000 for year one and a second year at another $100,000, provided that research milestones are achieved.

Our board members Roman Reed, Melissa King, Jason Cosgrove, and Darlene Brandenburg shared their excitement on AIM's social media sites and expressed their joy at seeing this three-month process develop in such a positive and meaningful way. Our entire team of AIM felt blessed to have received such excellent proposals and, in an irony of its own, we were truly honored to partner with UAB in our first round of research grant funding.

22

DESERVING PEACE

Home at last . . .
July 2014

With AIM's launch firmly under way, and as Ron and our family embraced a new year and a new chapter in our lives, I came to the conclusion that God had placed me in the right place, at the right time, doing what He had planned for me to do all along. In spite of the many personal challenges that had been thrown my way—my daughter Maggie's death, a traumatic divorce, personal sickness, loss of friendships, betrayals, and other disappointments—I saw that everything had led to this moment of being able to help people in a mighty way.

With many supporters, my children, my amazing husband Ron, and my best friend Roman Reed, we bolstered efforts for regenerative medicine research by creating the Alabama Institute of Medicine and three spin-off companies, all in less than two years. With the help of many, the AIM team is determined to change the scope of medicine by supporting cutting-edge stem cell treatments and cures in Alabama.

Roman and I feel blessed to have recruited a gifted team that fully shares the AIM mission. Our strength is the sum of these parts. And I think of the many thousands of people I pray our work will reach: a teenage girl with cancer, like my own sister, who hopes to resume a full life, of full health, just like Tera; a grandfather who wants to pitch to his grandson one more time before Parkinson's disease steals away the use of his body. I think of the young mother whose newborn has just been diagnosed with spinal muscular atrophy (SMA) and prays for movement, recovery, and healing. When I think of these precious faces, my concerns are replaced by courage, faith, and patience.

AIM is a reality, and it will lead us closer to discovering cures for disease and injury! In my abiding optimism that we will hopefully see profound changes and healing in my lifetime, I have to take a deep breath and remember that peace is part of God's plan. And wherever He leads, I will follow.

My favorite excerpt is from Matthew 6:

> That is why I am telling you not to worry about your life, and what you are to eat, nor about your body and what you are to wear. Surely life is more than food, and the body more than clothing! Can any of you, however much you worry, add one single cubit to your span of life? And why worry about clothing? Think of the flowers growing in the fields; they never have to work or spin; Yet I assure you that not even Solomon in all his royal robes was clothed like one of these. Now if that is how God clothes the wild flowers growing in the field . . . Will he not much more look after you, you who have so little faith? So do not worry; Do not say, "What are we to eat? What are we to drink? What are we to wear?" Your heavenly Father knows you need them all. Set your hearts on his kingdom first. . . . So do not worry about tomorrow: tomorrow will take care of itself. Each day has enough trouble of its own.

As this story closes—this journey and its inevitable collision of faith, love, loss, and life—I want to say thank-you for the many kind words and support I've received over these last few years. So many of you reading these words have traveled every step with me. I am here today because of your prayers and words of encouragement. Onwards and Upwards for Our Cures! Much love, ~ Tory

AFTERWORD

On September 10, 1994, my whole life changed. In a single second, I went from being one of America's best college football players to being paralyzed. I had once been able to bench press 430 pounds, until that moment. I was unable to move even my arms. I was only nineteen years old.

The doctor came into my hospital room and said, "Roman, I am sorry, but you will never move your arms and legs again or be able to father a child."

My reply, "Never tell me never! Get out of my room!"

I remember thinking I had a choice to make. I could leave this hospital in time, with my prescriptions and appointments for occupational therapy in my crippled hand. I could justify receiving disability checks from the government and slip away into a fog of painkillers and sleeping pills. But I wanted more out of life. My second option seemed extremely daunting but more like me, the fighter: paralysis would not define or beat me. I would do something about it, and help find cures for all. For me, the choice and path of my life was clear.

And so my journey for cures began.

Paralysis is a devastating condition that can be overwhelming for anyone, let alone a child suffering in a chair or bed for the rest of his or her life. How could I have looked at myself in the mirror if I had looked away from finding cures?

I quickly learned that in America we spend more on the annual care of our chronically injured than we bring in total federal income and corporate taxes COMBINED. That is unsustainable as a country. We can't pay for defense, education, or infrastructure without borrowing from other countries. Thus, I wanted to find cures not only for myself and my disabled brethren, but also for the fiscal sovereignty and well-being of our country.

After spending twenty years advocating and attending thousands of meetings with top researchers around the globe, I learned the importance and power of stem cells. Today, I understand that if we fully embrace this novel technology, we can move closer to curing the diseased and disabled like me. The economic effects of having our chronically injured go from receiving government checks to being fully employed and paying taxes to the government instead—this would be a fiscal boom almost beyond imagination. I know there are many people that care about curing the paralyzed, about giving their memories back to those with Alzheimer's, about curing cancer and extending lives. But with twenty-six states being led by legislatures that oppose this life-saving research, we must acknowledge that our science is under attack and take serious action to protect it.

My home state of California plans for another ten years of research funding through "CIRM 2," led again by my hero Robert Klein, who believes this is a way to tackle an ever-intensifying war on science. President Barack Obama might have loosened the restrictions on federal funding for embryonic stem cell research in 2009, but some presidential hopefuls—one of whom could be elected in 2016—support reinstating the Bush-era restrictions or even an outright ban on funding the work.

This is why I believe, through this story, Tory has the potential to reach millions and educate our world on the importance and power of stem cell research. And I know from working with her for over three years, that she has the heart, mind, and passion for this challenge.

Tory has come a long way since I first met her in 2011. She had not yet developed as an advocate and biotech leader. She had many concerns and zero confidence, but all of that would quickly change.

At first we conferred on everything. We had to, as she was a rookie earning her wings, and I had over fifteen years of experience and wisdom to guide her. But early on, she proved that her undivided heart was in this for the purest intent: the cause of cure. Tory took a firm grip on this challenge and stood against friends, family, coworkers, and employers who tried to silence her. She was told to either shut up or face severe consequences.

But for you and I, Tory would not be silenced in her advocacy and just blossomed from there. Thus, it soon got to the point that I could trust her to fly free, to be the light in the darkness that she truly is.

So today as I humbly write my contribution to this amazing story, I am honored to have been given this opportunity to partner with Tory on our law in Alabama, this book that many said would never become a reality, our beloved AIM that thrives with over $1.2 million in research dollars, and our newest venture, VivoStem.

It is my prayer that her name will go down in the laurels and history books of her beautiful state of Alabama and across the nation as a medical heroine who fought so passionately for physical and mental equality for all. And though some may try, no one can deny this, as I saw it firsthand.

Tory didn't have to reach out for my help three years ago, or to compromise herself and her family to pass a law bearing another's name. Regardless of the countless challenges she endured, Tory worked 24/7 to establish programs and foundations, and now to be a driving force behind several spin-off companies that will create jobs and improve her state's economy by advancing research and cures. Tory did all of this and so much more without ever asking once for anything in return. Not even the proceeds from this book are going into her pockets. Instead, Tory is pledging all to stem cell research and development, which is a commitment I have personally never witnessed. I am certain that God gave me Tory for this fight for cures, and I am optimistic that He will bless our efforts to help others.

Now moving forward, even closer toward our goals for cure, Tory and I hope that you will join us in this endeavor of spreading awareness and raising crucial funds for stem cell research. Just as actor Michael Douglas said while playing President Andrew Shepherd in the film *The American President*, "People don't drink the sand because they are thirsty, they drink the sand because they know no other way." Thus, when people are aware, there is no controversy.

An important fact to remember during your own advocacy for stem cell research: This technology does not destroy life; instead, stem cell research gives a deserving, independent life to those who are alive in spirit and mind but are dying on the inside from disease or injury.

Because I wear a lot of hats in my own relentless pursuit of cures, I am blessed that all of my positions meld into one that resonates my true purpose of life: my goal to contribute to a better life for all people. From being there to talk with a new paralyzed person to strategic stem cell alliance building, meeting with donors, keeping up with science updates and lab tours to being a social media fanatic, giving keynote speeches like my recent appearances at the World Stem Cell Summit and the National Neurotrauma Symposium, getting involved in local politics as planning commissioner and state politics as my recent campaign for state senate election, running my own foundation, helping pass a research law internationally with Perry Cross in Australia, and back to our great work in Alabama, which includes partnering with all of the states in the single and relentless pursuit of medical cures.

Most important, I am a doting father to three of the most amazing kids ever, named Roman Jr., Jason Troy, and my princess Katherine. And I am absolutely unequivocally certain that we will see stem cell cures in our lifetime. How many and how quickly are contingent upon funding and support of this research. I have given my life to this cause of making cures happen, and my life shall not be in vain.

I will walk again. You have my oath. And great people like you can help us reach this goal. Please take a stand for stem cell research, so that one day we can all stand together.

—Roman Reed

Acknowledgments

First and foremost, *Inevitable Collision* would not have been possible without the support of my family, friends, colleagues, and mentors mentioned throughout this story and on these final pages.

I want to thank my mother and father, who helped bring this book to you by encouraging me to write it. I am grateful to the two of them for their constant and unconditional love for as long as I can remember, and for all that they have taught me about empathy, the art of working around obstacles, and the importance of just getting the job done. I am grateful to them both for being wonderful role models to me, my siblings, and now, to their twelve grandchildren.

There will always be a special place in my heart for my sister Tera and my brother Brandon, who are my inspirations and whose love and support sustained me throughout.

As for my husband Ron, I find it difficult to express my appreciation because it is so boundless. He is my most enthusiastic cheerleader; he is my best friend; and he is an amazing husband and father to our seven children. He came into my life through the eye of the storm and calmed it to a beautiful sunset sky. With his gentle nudge and guidance, he taught me to stand up for myself and to never let anyone take advantage of my humility. Without his love and support, I would be lost.

And of course, my precious children, which includes four biological children and three stepchildren. It's hard to imagine this book being a reality without them. In fact, it is their bright smiles that put it all into perspective for me: Putting pen to paper to document this story and educate their generation on stem cell research is an important step in the right direction. But it's still not enough. To save this generation of children, we must build a stronger commitment from each arm of our state and federal government that will ensure safe and effective therapies reach our young and old without delay. My children remind me daily of all that is yet to be. Beyond this, I thank them for being so loving and patient during the months and years of research, writing, and editing, and for being such bundles of joy and laughter throughout the entire process.

A grateful heart to the best—and most patient—babysitter my children could have ever hoped for, McKinley Perry. We are so proud of McKinley and her many accomplishments and wish her all the best in pharmacy school and beyond.

I have been blessed to be surrounded by a loving and supportive extended family. A special thank-you to the Armstrong, Overstreet, and Williams family members who never wavered from their endless love and support before, during, and afterward.

From my years at Clarke-Washington EMC and time spent with fellow communication specialists across the state, I want to thank manager Stan Wilson for having faith in me as a writer and for giving me the opportunity to share with our readers the amazing stories of folks living in southwest Alabama. Chellie Phillips, Michael Cornelison, Suzanne Harrell, and Junior Carpenter just about had me convinced that I needed to stay at CWEMC forever.

And many thanks to Jason Boothe at the *Washington County News* and Jessica Ross of the Washington County Library who never once told me "No" if I asked for help with an article deadline, photo courtesy rights, or just to bounce around ideas—these two made the work-week a lot of fun.

I also owe a deep thank-you to Sandra Laton for encouraging me to pursue this project in the first place; Dana Massey, Tarah Olewski, and Dawn Hentz, who have been incredible friends to me over the years—their moral support has made all the difference; and Mrs. Lou Schell of

Chatom, author extraordinaire at the age of eighty-two, who inspired me to see this story through to publication no matter what obstacle may come my way.

Writing this book has also been a time of fantastic intellectual growth, fostered by a mix of wonderful learning environments from coast to coast beginning down south at the Shepherd Center, to Orange County, California's UC-Irvine, and all the way up the east coast to the Big Apple.

At Shepherd, the first person to whom I owe gratitude is Medical Director Dr. Donald Peck Leslie. There were numerous occasions when I felt disheartened and stumped about the direction of my research, but inevitably, a meeting with Dr. Leslie would reinvigorate my enthusiasm and raise my spirits immeasurably. He and his staff made my numerous visits to the center productive and meaningful experiences for this story.

There would be no clinical trial or a potential treatment for spinal cord injury had it not been for the hard work and tenacious spirit of Dr. Hans Keirstead at UC-Irvine. Hans has been a source of inspiration to me and many others through his research career and mentored thousands across the globe on the power and promise of stem cells. I still remember my first conversation with Hans, where he explained his ideology for research. "Tory," he said, "Always let the science lead." And this has been his mantra ever since. A special thanks to Hans for reviewing the early drafts of the science chapters and making excellent suggestions that transformed these hard-to-read pages into very understandable English for the non-PhDs like me.

I want to thank Dr. Paul Knoepfler at UC-Davis and Dr. Edward Wirth and Dr. Jane Lebkowski from Asterias Biotherapeutics, Inc., whose dedication to the research field is incredible. No acknowledgement can truly express how grateful Roman and I are to have gained their friendship and advice over the years.

Two other researchers who have had an important influence on me are UAB's Dr. Timothy Wick and Dr. Joanne Murphy-Ullrich. They have both been wonderful collaborators and generous friends to our nonprofit program AIM. I have learned a lot about clinical research through my involvement and friendship with them.

On the East Coast, I want to thank Brooke Ellison for being a hero to me and millions more. Brooke, a champion advocate for stem cell research, was among the first to offer support of our efforts in the Deep

South. And many thanks to the brilliant producer Todd Leatherman for sharing his passion for life and bringing awareness to all that our world encompasses. To David McKeon of the New York Stem Cell Foundation, I wish to say thank-you for your generosity during my visit to the NYSCF, and for the kind email sent to Bernie Siegel following our meeting.

An endless thanks to Susan Leon, a twenty-five-year-experienced editor and manuscript evaluator, for believing in me and reaffirming that I had an important story to share with the public. You enabled me to muster enough courage to translate my thoughts and ideas that formed this book, and I will forever be grateful for your hard work, patience, and editorial advice on this project.

A big thank-you to Jayne Woolf, Jennifer Quigley, Larry Bernstein, and the entire Mary Ann Liebert Publishing Team. I couldn't have done this without you. And many thanks to our wonderful PR team, Melanie Scharler and Mara Wedeck, also known as the dynamic duo M&M.

To Vivo Biosciences, Inc., for providing the financial sponsorship for this book. Your support made everything possible. I have been touched and honored to work with the VBI team in this partnership for cures.

Thanks to AIM's board of directors, Darlene Brandenburg, Jason Cosgrove, and Melissa King, who have given a tremendous amount of time and energy to advance stem cell research in Alabama. Your wisdom, leadership, and commitment to AIM inspires us all.

And last, but definitely first, I want to thank my mentor and great friend Roman Reed, not just because he has given up so much to make medical care and cures a priority in our lives, but also because he has seen me through the ups and downs of the entire advocacy and writing process. Roman has shared this amazing journey with me, so it only seems right that I dedicate this book to him.

Onwards and Upwards, always.
God bless!
~Tory

Index